Chronic Total Occlusion

Guest Editor

WILLIAM L. LOMBARDI, MD

INTERVENTIONAL CARDIOLOGY CLINICS

www.interventional.theclinics.com

Consulting Editors
SAMIN K. SHARMA, MD
IGOR F. PALACIOS, MD

July 2012 • Volume 1 • Number 3

SAUNDERS an imprint of ELSEVIER, Inc.

W.B. SAUNDERS COMPANY
A Division of Elsevier Inc.

1600 John F. Kennedy Boulevard • Suite 1800 • Philadelphia, Pennsylvania 19103-2899

http://www.theclinics.com

INTERVENTIONAL CARDIOLOGY CLINICS Volume 1, Number 3
July 2012 ISSN 2211-7458, ISBN-13: 978-1-4557-4893-8

Editor: Barbara Cohen-Kligerman
Developmental Editor: Teia Stone

Interventional Cardiology Clinics (ISSN 2211-7458) is published quarterly by Elsevier Inc., 360 Park Avenue South, New York, NY 10010-1710. Months of issue are January, April, July, and October. Subscription prices are USD 177 per year for US individuals, USD 119 per year for US students, USD 265 per year for Canadian individuals, USD 129 per year for Canadian students, USD 265 per year for international individuals, and USD 136 per year for international students. To receive student/resident rate, orders must be accompanied by name of affiliated institution, date of term, and the *signature* of program/residency coordinator on institution letterhead. Orders will be billed at individual rate until proof of status is received. Foreign air speed delivery is included in all *Clinics* subscription prices. All prices are subject to change without notice. **POSTMASTER:** Send address changes to *Interventional Cardiology Clinics*, Elsevier Health Sciences Division, Subscription Customer Service, 3251 Riverport Lane, Maryland Heights, MO 63043. **Customer Service:** Telephone: 1-800-654-2452 (U.S. and Canada); **1-314-447-8871** (outside U.S. and Canada). **Fax: 1-314-447-8029.** E-mail: **journalscustomerservice-usa@elsevier.com** (for print support); **journalsonlinesupport-usa@ elsevier.com** (for online support).

Reprints. For copies of 100 or more of articles in this publication, please contact the Commercial Reprints Department, Elsevier Inc., 360 Park Avenue South, New York, NY 10010-1710. Tel.: 212-633-3812; Fax: 212-462-1935; E-mail: reprints@elsevier.com.

Printed and bound by CPI Group (UK) Ltd, Croydon, CR0 4YY

Transferred to Digital Print 2012

Contributors

CONSULTING EDITORS

SAMIN K. SHARMA, MD, FSCAI, FACC
Director of Clinical Cardiology; Director of
Cardiac Catheterization Laboratory, Mount
Sinai Medical Center, New York, New York

IGOR F. PALACIOS, MD, FSCAI
Director of Interventional Cardiology,
Cardiology Division, Heart Center,
Massachusetts General Hospital; Associate
Professor of Medicine, Harvard Medical
School, Boston, Massachusetts

GUEST EDITOR

WILLIAM L. LOMBARDI, MD, FACC, FSCAI
Cardiac Catheterization Laboratory Director,
PeaceHealth St. Joseph Medical Center,
Bellingham, Washington

AUTHORS

KHALDOON ALASWAD, MD, RVT, FACC, FSCAI, FSVM
Director, Catheterization Laboratory, Appleton
Heart Institute, Appleton, Wisconsin

RODRIGO BAGUR, MD
Interventional Cardiology Laboratories,
Quebec Heart & Lung Institute—Laval
University, Québec (Québec), Canada

SUBHASH BANERJEE, MD
Division of Cardiology, VA North Texas Health
Care System, The University of Texas
Southwestern Medical Center at Dallas,
Dallas, Texas

EMMANOUIL S. BRILAKIS, MD, PhD
Director, Cardiac Catheterization Laboratory,
Division of Cardiology, VA North Texas Health
Care System, The University of Texas
Southwestern Medical Center at Dallas,
Dallas, Texas

M. NICHOLAS BURKE, MD, FSCAI
Senior Consulting Cardiologist, Minneapolis
Heart Institute and Foundation, Minneapolis,
Minnesota

TONY J. DEMARTINI, MD
Clinical Assistant Professor of Medicine,
Southern Illinois University School of Medicine;
Prairie Cardiovascular Consultants,
Springfield, Illinois

SUDHAKAR GIROTRA, MD
Department of Interventional Cardiology,
Banner Good Samaritan Medical Center,
Phoenix, Arizona

J. AARON GRANTHAM, MD, FACC
Associate Professor of Medicine, University of
Missouri-Kansas City, Saint Luke's Mid
America Heart Institute, Kansas City, Missouri

DAVID E. KANDZARI, MD, FACC, FSCAI
Chief Scientific Officer and Director,
Interventional Cardiology, Piedmont Heart
Institute, Atlanta, Georgia

DIMITRI KARMPALIOTIS, MD, FACC
Interventional Cardiology, Piedmont Heart
Institute, Atlanta, Georgia

EVAN LAU, MD
Interventional Cardiology Fellow, Robert
and Suzanne Tomsich Department of
Cardiovascular Medicine, Cleveland Clinic
Foundation, Cleveland, Ohio

NICHOLAS J. LEMBO, MD, FACC, FSCAI
Medical Director, Coronary Therapeutics
Center of Excellence, Piedmont Heart Institute,
Atlanta, Georgia

VISHAL PATEL, MD
Division of Cardiology, VA North Texas Health
Care System, The University of Texas
Southwestern Medical Center at Dallas,
Dallas, Texas

ASHISH PERSHAD, MD, FACC, FSCAI
Department of Interventional Cardiology,
Banner Good Samaritan Medical Center,
Phoenix, Arizona

STÉPHANE RINFRET, MD, SM, FRCP(C)
Interventional Cardiology Laboratories,
Quebec Heart & Lung Institute—Laval
University, Québec (Québec), Canada

RIMON L. SHAKER, MD
Department of Interventional Cardiology,
Banner Good Samaritan Medical Center,
Phoenix, Arizona

JAMES C. SPRATT, MD, FRCP, FESC, FACC
Consultant Cardiologist, Department of
Cardiology, Forth Valley Royal Hospital,
Larbert, United Kingdom

JULIAN W. STRANGE, MBChB, MD, FRCP
Consultant Cardiologist, Bristol Heart Institute,
University Hospitals Bristol NHS Foundation
Trust, Bristol, United Kingdom

CRAIG A. THOMPSON, MD, MMSc
Director, Cardiovascular Catheterization and
Intervention, Yale New Haven Hospital, Yale
University School of Medicine, New Haven,
Connecticut

KETHES C. WARAM, MD
Department of Interventional Cardiology,
Banner Good Samaritan Medical Center,
Phoenix, Arizona

PATRICK WHITLOW, MD
Director of Interventional Cardiology, Robert
and Suzanne Tomsich Department of
Cardiovascular Medicine, Cleveland Clinic
Foundation, Cleveland, Ohio

NICHOLAS P. WILLIS, MD
Department of Interventional Cardiology,
Banner Good Samaritan Medical Center,
Phoenix, Arizona

R. MICHAEL WYMAN, MD, FACC
Director, Cardiovascular Interventional
Research, Torrance Memorial Medical
Center, Torrance, California

Contents

Chronic total occlusion accounts for 15% of cases during diagnostic angiography with higher referral rate to surgical revascularization. With contemporary strategies and techniques, the success rate with experienced operators can exceed 90%. Currently available observational studies in carefully selected patient populations show evidence of a trend toward symptom relief; improvement in quality of life, left ventricular function, and mortality; and improved tolerance toward future ischemic events. Lack of randomized controlled trials comparing current optimal medical management with percutaneous coronary intervention for chronic total occlusion is a major barrier to widespread adaptation of this advanced complex interventional technique.

More interventional cardiologists are adopting chronic total occlusion (CTO) percutaneous coronary intervention (PCI) in their practice. This article follows the steps of the PCI procedure to describe the toolbox and inventory requirements for successful program development. Recent innovations have allowed adoption of controlled dissection and reentry techniques as a primary revascularization strategy for CTO. Other devices have special rules in CTO PCI. Equipment and techniques to enhance guide catheter support are frequently needed during CTO PCI. Tools for complication management are important components. The necessary tools are listed at the end of the article.

Chronic total occlusion percutaneous coronary intervention (CTO PCI) procedural planning involves much thought and deliberation before one actually attempts to cross the CTO lesion in the cardiac catheterization laboratory. Careful preprocedural angiographic assessment is a key to successful CTO PCI. CTO PCI represents the most complex PCI one can perform, and thus operator and staff training as well as the concept of CTO days are all essential for a successful CTO PCI program.

This article discusses interventional guidewires in general and how they are best used in chronic total occlusion (CTO) percutaneous coronary intervention (PCI) in particular. The components that make a guidewire and the various design options are described. The specific characteristics of these options and how they relate to various aspects of PCI are discussed. Guidewire design as it applies specifically to the tasks particular to CTO PCI is discussed.

Over the last two decades, the transradial approach has gained an important role in interventional cardiology. A large body of evidence exists supporting the safety and feasibility of the transradial approach in a broad spectrum of patients and settings. In addition, the transradial approach has been applied with good results for chronic total occlusion (CTO) recanalization. This article provides an overview of basic principles and techniques required to perform successful transradial CTO percutaneous coronary intervention.

This article focuses on the general principles of informed consent, then highlights the particular risks associated with chronic total occlusion interventions. The goal is to provide a basic framework for the interventional cardiologist to use when having consent discussions with his or her patients.

Every percutaneous coronary intervention carries risk for acute and long-term complications. This is also true of chronic total occlusion (CTO) interventions, which can also have complications specific to specialized techniques, such as retrograde crossing and dissection/reentry techniques. Acute CTO intervention complications can be coronary artery–related, cardiac noncoronary, or noncardiac. In the long term, CTO interventions can be complicated by in-stent restenosis, stent thrombosis, or coronary aneurysm formation. Understanding of the pathogenesis of possible CTO intervention complications can facilitate prevention, early recognition, and prompt treatment.

Against the background of current data supporting indications for chronic total occlusion (CTO) revascularization and strategies that promote incrementally higher procedural success rates, this article introduces a multidisciplinary approach to CTO program development, establishes guidelines for the performance of safe and efficient CTO percutaneous coronary intervention, and reviews considerations related to resource utilization and economic outcomes with complex percutaneous coronary revascularization.

INTERVENTIONAL CARDIOLOGY CLINICS

Preface

The Final Frontier of Percutaneous Coronary Intervention—Coronary Chronic Total Occlusions

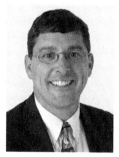

William L. Lombardi, MD
Guest Editor

This issue of *Interventional Cardiology Clinics* goes in depth into the final frontier of percutaneous coronary intervention, coronary chronic total occlusions (CTOs). Historically, CTOs have been the most difficult lesions to be treated by percutaneous techniques. In addition, CTOs have been the biggest predictor of patients being referred for coronary artery bypass surgery, incomplete revascularization, mortality after ST elevation myocardial infarction, and mortality after non-ST myocardial infarction. A multitude of reasons exists for failure of percutaneous techniques to conquer these challenging lesions, but as will be revealed in the following articles, many of those historical barriers have been removed. As you read through these articles, you will learn that many of your colleagues have already mastered the new techniques and will share those with you.

Over the course of this issue you will learn the indications for coronary CTO revascularization with an emphasis not just on CTO but on the importance of reducing ischemic burden. You will become acquainted with the parsimonious toolbox, which will guide you to having the right equipment in your cath lab to be successful. The complex techniques are broken down into their parts for you to learn that in reality these procedures can be predictable if you evolve from an interventionalist to a CTO interventionalist. Dr Thompson shows that once you have learned the skill sets for CTO revascularization, a straightforward algorithm for anatomic decision-making can improve success and efficiency. We then discuss the nuances of consent to and complications of these procedures. Last, how to build a successful program and the financial benefits to your institution are covered.

The final frontier has been crossed by a multitude of interventional cardiologists. The anatomy of a CTO has been removed as a predictor of success and should not be used to determine clinical relevance. Given the number of centers that have already developed successful and efficient programs, readers need to consider whether they will also develop the skill set to build a successful program. The challenge I pose to the reader is, are you going to be leading the way in developing this skill set or will you be the last? After you have read the articles in this issue, I hope you will join your colleagues at www.ctofundamentals.org

Intervent Cardiol Clin 1 (2012) ix–x
doi:10.1016/j.iccl.2012.05.002

a web site dedicated to educating physicians on CTO percutaneous intervention. Many resources are available to help you achieve the proficiency that allows you to conquer CTOs. In conclusion, I would like to welcome you to the final frontier of coronary intervention and wish you luck in developing this skill set.

William L. Lombardi, MD
PeaceHealth St. Joseph Medical Center
2979 Squalicom Parkway, Suite 101
Bellingham, WA 98225, USA

E-mail address:
WLombardi@peacehealth.org

Rationale for Percutaneous Intervention of CTO

Kethes C. Waram, MD, Nicholas P. Willis, MD,
Sudhakar Girotra, MD, Rimon L. Shaker, MD,
Ashish Pershad, MD*

KEYWORDS

- Chronic total occlusion • Indication for CTO • Mortality • Myocardial perfusion • Clinical outcome

KEY POINTS

- Chronic total occlusion (CTO) accounts for 15% of cases during diagnostic angiography with a higher referral rate for surgical revascularization.
- With contemporary strategies and techniques, the success rate with experienced operators can exceed 90%.
- Currently available observational studies in carefully selected patient populations show evidence of a trend toward symptom relief; improvement in quality of life (QOL), left ventricular (LV) function, and a mortality benefit; and an improved tolerance of future ischemic events.
- Lack of randomized controlled trials comparing current optimal medical management with percutaneous coronary intervention (PCI) for CTO is a major barrier to widespread adoption of this advanced complex interventional technique.

I would have every man write what he knows and no more.

—*Montaigne*

INTRODUCTION

CTO is characterized by coronary artery compromise that results in complete interruption of antegrade blood flow. In the absence of serial angiograms, the duration of coronary occlusions is difficult to specify but an occlusion of greater than 90 days is considered chronic by unanimity. Most occlusion durations are estimated from available clinical information related to the timing of the event that caused the occlusion (eg, acute myocardial infarction [MI] or change in angina pattern). The true prevalence of CTO remains unknown because large percentages of patients are asymptomatic or minimally symptomatic and never undergo diagnostic angiography.

CTO PCI is the last frontier in coronary intervention.[1] It is the most common reason for referral of patients with multivessel coronary artery disease for coronary artery bypass graft (CABG).[2] In the United States, contemporary attempt rates are in the 11% to 15% range. Even high-volume PCI operators attempt approximately only 20% of CTOs they encounter.[3]

Why has CTO PCI not gained widespread acceptance and adoption? The absence of a randomized controlled trial demonstrating superiority of PCI over best contemporary medical therapy has been the biggest barrier to widespread adoption. Operator inexperience and reluctance to embark on time-intensive, resource-intensive, and complex procedures with potential complications, including vessel perforation, radiation injury, contrast nephropathy, and loss of native coronary collaterals, are other barriers.[3] There is a misperception that the Occluded Artery Trial's[4] lack of reduction in clinical events after routine PCI in stable patients with totally occluded infarct-related arteries (IRAs) after the subacute phase of an MI is applicable to the

Department of Interventional Cardiology, Banner Good Samaritan Medical Center, 1111 East McDowell Road, Phoenix, AZ 85006, USA
* Corresponding author. 1331 North 7th Street, Suite 375, Phoenix, AZ 85006.
E-mail address: asper1971@gmail.com

Intervent Cardiol Clin 1 (2012) 265–279
doi:10.1016/j.iccl.2012.04.003

interventional.theclinics.com

CTO population. The key differentiating factor is that the myocardium subtended by the IRAs in Occluded Artery Trial patients are recently infarcted in contrast to CTO cases where the myocardium is viable at various stages of the ischemic cascade depending on the natural history.

Other misconceptions include the idea that the territory subtended by the occluded artery is well collateralized and, therefore, not ischemic; the vessel is already occluded and no further damage or harm can occur, implying a stable coronary lesion subset. These reasons are used as justification for either medically treating CTO lesions or, in the setting of multivessel disease, referring patients to CABG and avoiding an attempt at PCI. Limited insights into or uncertainty of the benefits of CTO recanalization to patients' overall health status has contributed to the reluctance of society guideline committees to favorably recommend PCI. This translates into further underutilization of PCI for CTO.

PATHOBIOLOGY

Although the histopathology of the chronically occluded coronary artery has been comprehensively described,[5,6] there remains much to learn about the various stages and natural evaluation of the occlusion (**Fig. 1**).[7] Chronic coronary occlusions most often arise from thrombotic occlusion, followed by thrombus organization and tissue aging with varying degrees of recanalization. This article systematically reviews the literature and attempts to answer the question, What is the rationale for PCI of CTOs? In an era where evidence-based medicine reigns, intellectual honesty must be enforced in treating all lesion subsets, including CTOs.

REVIEW

The rationale for treatment of any coronary stenosis starts with identifying the right patients. The 5 principal reasons for attempting to open a CTO are listed in **Box 1**.

POTENTIAL MORTALITY BENEFIT

The earliest article that demonstrated mortality benefit was by Suero and colleagues,[8] during the era of balloon angioplasty. This remains the single largest observational series, with more than 2000 patients followed for more than 10 years, which provides great insights regarding CTO PCI. Patients who underwent unsuccessful single-vessel CTO procedure derived mortality benefit, even when their CTO was surgically bypassed, compared with medical therapy (71.2% vs 63.9%). This provided proof of concept that treatment of CTOs,

whether by angioplasty or bypass, was successful in providing a mortality benefit. Another key finding of this study was that, despite the perception that CTO intervention carries inherent increased procedure-related risk relative to non-CTO interventions, the 10-year survival rate was not different between these 2 groups (73.5% vs 71.9%; $P = .33$) (**Fig. 2**). This study also demonstrated that CTO in patients represent a spectrum or continuum of coronary artery disease, with the best outcomes occurring in patients with single-vessel CTO and successful recanalization. At the other end of the spectrum, the worst outcomes occurred in patients with CTO who also had multivessel disease and had unsuccessful recanalization.

The Total Occlusion Angioplasty Study supported by Societá Italiana di Cardiologia Invasiva (TOAST-GISE)[9] was a prospective multicenter study from Italy that included 376 patients with CTO followed for a 1-year period. The technical success for percutaneous recanalization was 77%, but the definition of CTO included an artery was occluded more than 30 days, not the traditional definition of more than 90 days. The investigators reported fewer cardiac deaths in the successfully treated group compared with those with a failed procedure. Although the actual number of cardiac deaths reported was small (n = 4), the difference between the 2 groups was statistically significant ($P = .037$). Limitations include the small number of patients enrolled, rates of PCI performed in non-CTO arteries not reported, and only patients discharged from the hospital free of major adverse cardiac events (MACE) included in the survival analysis.

In the 10-year experience of the Thoraxcenter at the Erasmus MC,[10] 874 consecutive patients treated for CTO were followed for a median duration of 4.48 years with excellent long-term follow-up. In the retrospective observational analysis, the cumulative survival at 5 years was 88% in the group in which the CTO was unsuccessfully treated versus 93.5% in the group whose CTO was treated successfully (hazard ratio [HR] 0.58; 95% CI, 0.34–0.98). The survival benefit was most apparent in those with multivessel disease and was unaffected by the diabetic status of the population. In this study, the propensity model was not adjusted for the extent of revascularization performed or adjunctive medications, which may represent limitations of this study.

In the Mayo Clinic experience of 1262 patients, Prasad and colleagues[11] demonstrated that successful PCI of a CTO conferred a mortality benefit when compared with an unsuccessful attempt. This mortality benefit did not manifest until 6 years into the follow-up but was statistically

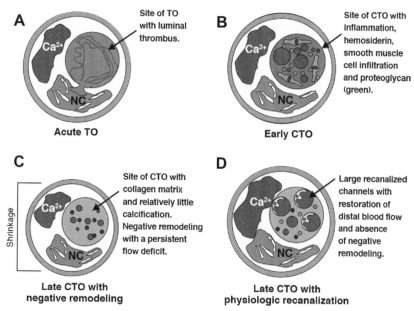

Fig. 1. Morphologic characteristics of CTO. (*A*) Acute plaque rupture is shown, with luminal thrombus resulting in CTO. (*B*) Inflammation with early thrombus organization is shown. Note early recanalization accompanied by proteoglycan matrix (green) in the area of total occlusion (TO). (*C*) The late chronic phase of healed TO is shown, with deposition of collagen type I where the cross-linking of collagen promotes negative remodeling of the vessel. (*D*) Physiologic recanalization is accompanied by restoration of normal flow distally, thus preventing negative remodeling. (*From* Finn AV, Kolodgie FD, Nakano M, et al. The differences between neovascularization of chronic total occlusion and intraplaque angiogenesis. JACC Cardiovasc Imaging 2010;3(8):806–10; with permission.)

significant (*P* = .025). After adjustment for patient characteristics, there was a 4% relative risk reduction in mortality per year after 6 years in the group with successful CTO recanalization versus the group with unsuccessful recanalization (**Fig. 3**). Aziz and colleagues[12] reported a retrospective observational study of 400 CTO lesions with a primary endpoint of mortality at 2 years. In this study, an unsuccessful attempt at CTO recanalization resulted in an HR of 4.95 (95% CI, 1.03–23.89). The small number of patients with hard endpoints limits the validity of the Cox proportional hazards model but the mortality benefit held true for both single-vessel and multivessel disease patients. Valenti and colleagues[13] published their data on

486 patients in which a mortality benefit was demonstrated over a 2-year follow-up in patients with successful CTO recanalization. In this study, patients with successful CTO recanalization had a survival rate of 91.4% at 2 years versus 86.6% in those with unsuccessful CTO recanalization (*P* = .02) (**Fig. 4**). In addition, this study showed a survival benefit in those with complete revascularization versus those with incomplete revascularization (94% vs 83.8% survival at 2 years; *P*<.001) (**Fig. 5**). The limitation of this trial lies in the incompleteness of data related to medical therapy.

Safley and colleagues[14] demonstrated that single-vessel CTO revascularization of the left anterior descending artery, but not the left circumflex or the right coronary artery (RCA), was independently predictive of survival at 5 years, with an HR of 0.61 (95% CI, 0.42–0.89). Their survival model was not adjusted for key mortality predictors, such as renal insufficiency, LV ejection fraction (LVEF), and baseline medications. This serves as a limitation in the validity of the conclusions reached by the investigators.

There have been studies that failed to demonstrate mortality benefit from CTO revascularization. The first was by Lee and colleagues[15] from Korea in which there were methodologic flaws and a small number of patients. The primary endpoint was a combined MACE at 2 years, which included death, cardiovascular death, MI, and

---

Box 1

Five main reasons for attempting to open a CTO

1. Potential for mortality benefit after successful revascularization

2. Relief of angina

3. Improvement in ischemic burden in asymptomatic patients or those with minimal symptoms

4. Improvement in LV function

5. Improved tolerance for future ischemic events

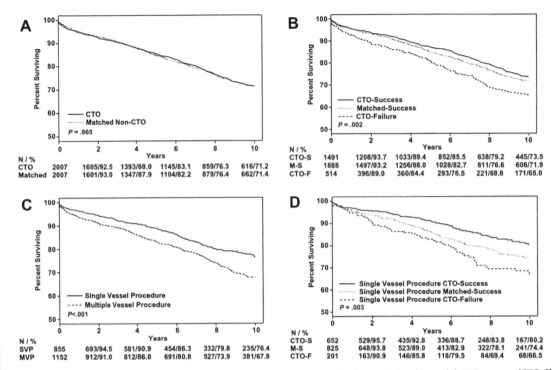

Fig. 2. Cumulative 10-year survival. (*A*) Chronic total CTO versus matched non-CTO cohorts. (*B*) CTO success (CTO-S) versus matched non-CTO success (M-S) versus CTO failure (CTO-F) groups. (*C*) Single-vessel procedure (SVP) versus multivessel procedure (MVP). (*D*) SVP CTO-S versus SVP-matched M-S versus SVP CTO-F. (*From* Suero JA, Marso SP, Jones PG, et al. Procedural outcomes and long term survival among patients undergoing percutaneous coronary intervention of a chronic total occlusion in native coronary arteries: a 20 year experience. J Am Coll Cardiol 2001;38(2):409–14; with permission.)

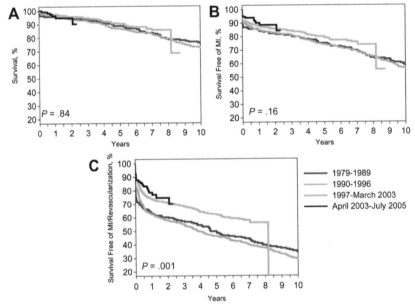

Fig. 3. Kaplan-Meier estimates for (*A*) death, (*B*) death or MI, and (*C*) death, MI, or target lesion revascularzation in the 4 groups. The sudden survival decrease at approximately 8 years for the 1997 to March 2003 group was the result of an event occurring among a few patients still at risk and reflects the instability of the estimator when few patients remain. The curves are presented to 10 years, however, for the benefit of comparing the 10-year estimates of the 2 earliest groups. (*From* Prasad A, Rihal CS, Lennon RJ, et al. Trends in outcomes after percutaneous coronary intervention for chronic total occlusions: a 25 year experience from the Mayo Clinic. J Am Coll Cardiol 2007;49:1611–8; with permission.)

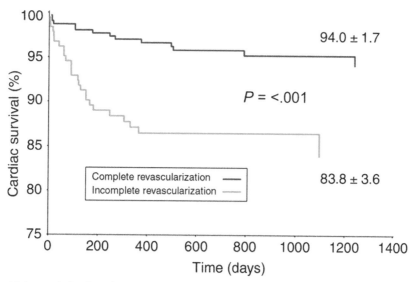

Fig. 4. Kaplan-Meier analysis of cardiac survival in patients with complete revascularization when compared with patients with incomplete revascularization. (*From* Valenti R, Migliorini A, Signorini U, et al. Impact of complete revascularization with percutaneous coronary intervention on survival in patients with at least one chronic total occlusion. Eur Heart J 2008;29(19):2336–42; with permission.)

target vessel revascularization. In the unsuccessful CTO group, failure to include those patients who went to CABG after a failed attempt at revascularization was a weakness of the study. Those 7 patients were discarded from the statistical analysis. This made outcomes in the unsuccessful CTO group look much better. If these patients had been included in the statistical analysis, the results would have been different.

Investigators from the Washington Hospital Center[16] published their experience in 172 patients with 2-year follow-up. They concluded that there was no difference in mortality at 2 years in

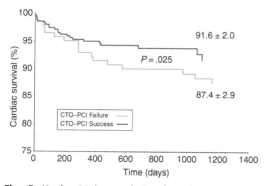

Fig. 5. Kaplan-Meier analysis of cardiac survival in patients with CTO PCI success compared with patients with CTO PCI failure. (*From* Valenti R, Migliorini A, Signorini U, et al. Impact of complete revascularization with percutaneous coronary intervention on survival in patients with at least one chronic total occlusion. Eur Heart J 2008;29(19):2336–42; with permission.)

patients with and without successful CTO recanalization (5.3% vs 4.9%). A major limitation of this study was that they excluded patients with major procedural complications and their propensity analysis was unadjusted.

A major limitation of all the studies discussed previously is that they excluded patients in whom CTO recanalization was not attempted for various reasons, including lack of symptoms, complex angiographic features, or significant comorbidities. This selection bias can account for a significant α error. If a prospective randomized controlled trial is performed with all-cause mortality and cardiovascular mortality as a primary endpoint, only then can the question of mortality benefit with CTO revascularization be answered. Data obtained from meta-analysis, however, such as in Joyal and colleagues' study,[17] and from single-center series cannot be discarded because the preponderance of studies have shown a mortality benefit (**Fig. 6**).

The mechanisms associated with increased survival in patients with successful recanalization of CTOs are not completely clear. One theory is that collateral circulation leads to chronically hibernating but viable myocardium, which when more adequately perfused leads to mortality benefit due to decreased sudden cardiac death or less adverse cardiac remodeling. Also there is the possibility that a clinical subset of patients have improved survival after CTO recanalization, such as patients with left main disease and an accompanying CTO of RCA or diabetics because of their

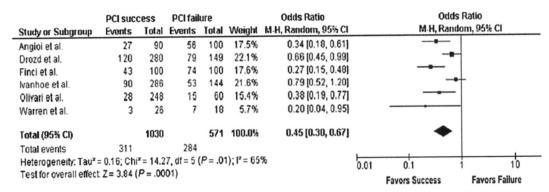

Study or Subgroup	PCI success Events	Total	PCI failure Events	Total	Weight	Odds Ratio M-H, Random, 95% CI	Odds Ratio M-H, Random, 95% CI
Angioi et al.	27	90	56	100	17.5%	0.34 [0.18, 0.61]	
Drozd et al.	120	280	79	149	22.1%	0.66 [0.45, 0.99]	
Finci et al.	43	100	74	100	17.6%	0.27 [0.15, 0.48]	
Ivanhoe et al.	90	286	53	144	21.6%	0.79 [0.52, 1.20]	
Olivari et al.	28	248	15	60	15.4%	0.38 [0.19, 0.77]	
Warren et al.	3	26	7	18	5.7%	0.20 [0.04, 0.95]	
Total (95% CI)		1030		571	100.0%	0.45 [0.30, 0.67]	
Total events	311		284				

Heterogeneity: Tau² = 0.16; Chi² = 14.27, df = 5 (P = .01); I² = 65%
Test for overall effect: Z = 3.84 (P = .0001)

Favors Success   Favors Failure

Fig. 6. Effect of successful versus failed CTO recanalization on all-cause mortality during available follow-up. Odds ratio of mortality benefit in all CTO series. (*From* Joyal D, Afilalo J, Rinfret S. Effectiveness of recanalization of chronic total occlusions: a systematic review and meta-analysis. Am Heart J 2010;160(1):179–87; with permission.)

less robust collaterals. This remains an area of active research and future investigation.

ANGINA RELIEF WITH CTO REVASCULARIZATION

Stable angina is the most common presentation of symptomatic patients with CTOs. Recanalization of CTOs for the purpose of relieving anginal symptoms has long been recognized as a rationale for PCI. The Stable Angina Pectoris Registry[18] showed that approximately one-third of patients undergoing angiography for stable angina had at least one CTO. Recanalization of CTO using plain old balloon angioplasty was shown to have a benefit in reduction of angina. Ruocco and colleagues[19] found similar improvement in angina class after percutaneous transluminal coronary angioplasty (PTCA) between patients who had total and subtotal coronary occlusions. Their review of the National Heart, Lung, and Blood Institute angioplasty registry from 1985 to 1986 reported that 94% of patients with single-vessel CTO had either no angina or improvement of their symptoms at 2 years after successful recanalization, similar to the 92% of patients who reported symptom improvement after successful PTCA for a subtotal occlusion. Likewise, in patients undergoing PTCA for multiple stenoses, 92% of those with at least one CTO had either no angina or reduced symptoms at 2 years after successful intervention versus 94% of patients having angina improvement in the subtotal occlusion cohort.

Bell and colleagues[20] analyzed patients between 1979 and 1990 who had attempted PTCA to CTOs. They found no significant difference between the 2 groups with respect to angina burden during follow-up. There were significantly more patients requiring CABG, however, after a failed procedure versus a successful recanalization (P<.0001) **(Fig. 7)**. Noguchi and colleagues[21] found similar

results when analyzing 226 consecutive patients undergoing attempted PTCA to CTO. Both studies, in addition to showing increased need for CABG after a failed recanalization of a CTO, also showed that the need for surgical revascularization occurred early after the failed percutaneous procedure, implicating persistent anginal symptoms as the driver for the need for CABG.

Despite the aforementioned studies in which angina relief was substantially higher in patients with successful CTO recanalization versus those in which CTO revascularization was unsuccessful, there remains a large amount of skepticism because the studies were in the balloon angioplasty or bare metal stent era when restenosis and reocclusion were both high and the success rates were 60% to 65%. Two contemporary trials have attempted to systematically look at this

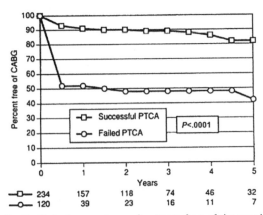

Fig. 7. Plot of percentage of patients free of the need for CABG surgery according to the outcome of initial angioplasty. (*From* Bell MR, Berger PB, Bresnahan JF, et al. Initial and long-term outcome of 354 patients after coronary balloon angioplasty of total coronary artery occlusions. Circulation 1992;85(3):1003–11; with permission.)

subject. The first was a single-center prospective cohort analysis performed in the UK. The investigators looked at changes in angina frequency and perception using a specific questionnaire on angina-related QOL (Seattle Angina Questionnaire [SAQ]-UK version).[22] This questionnaire consists of 14 items that assess 3 dimensions of angina: (1) physical activity limitation, (2) angina frequency and perception, and (3) treatment satisfaction. The validity and reliability of this questionnaire has been previously demonstrated. Seventy percent of the 302 patients who participated in the study[23] answered the angina questionnaire. The procedural success rate was 78% and in-hospital complication rate was 3%. The complication rate was no different between the 2 groups. The median follow-up was for 4 years. Patients with a failed attempt had a higher risk of cardiac death (HR 3.39; $P = .03$) after propensity score adjustment compared with those who had a successful procedure. Patients with successful revascularization had less physical activity limitation, rarer angina episodes, and greater patient satisfaction compared with patients with a failed procedure ($P<.03$ for all 3 components) with improved overall acceptable quality level scores (**Table 1**).

The second contemporary trial that systematically evaluated QOL with the SAQ was the FlowCardia Approach to CTO Recanalization (FACTOR) trial.[24] A total of 125 patients completed the SAQ at baseline and 1 month after CTO PCI.

One-month health status outcomes were compared by multivariable analysis, adjusting for group differences between those whose CTO was successfully recanalized and those unsuccessfully recanalized (**Fig. 8**). Procedural success was 55% (n = 64) and independently associated with angina relief (difference between those with successful and unsuccessful PCI [Δ] in SAQ angina frequency = 9.5 points [95% CI, 1.6–17.5; $P = .019$], improved physical function [Δ in SAQ physical limitation = 13.1 points; 95% CI, 5.1–21.1; $P = .001$], and enhanced QOL [Δ in SAQ QOL = 20.3 points; 95% CI, 11.9–28.6; $P<.001$]). The benefit of successful PCI was greatest in patients who were symptomatic at baseline compared with asymptomatic patients although statistically significantly only for QOL (ΔSAQ angina frequency domain = 10.3 vs 4.3 points, $P = .51$; Δ physical limitation = 15.9 vs 6.3 points, $P = .25$; and Δ QOL = 27.3 vs 8.5 points, $P = .047$).

IMPROVEMENT IN LV FUNCTION

It is a challenge to identify the right patients who might benefit from revascularization of a CTO. Simple methods, such as the absence of Q waves on an EKG or the absence of a history of a prior MI, to advanced imaging, such as positron emission tomography (PET) and cardiac MRI, have been used to predict which patients might have LV function improvement after revascularization. Sirnes

Table 1
SAQ scores and CCS functional class after CTO procedure and changes versus preprocedure in patients with essential and failed CTO recanalization

SAQ-UK	Successful CTO Treatment	Failed CTO Treatment	P Value
Physical limitation (%)	82.2	70.9	.01
Change vs preprocedure	+28.1	+16.7	.01
Angina frequency (%)	81.6	55.0	<.001
Change vs preprocedure	+29.1	−9.2	<.001
Rx satisfaction	89.2	80.0	.03
CCS class			
Asymptomatic (%)	53.1	30.5	<.001
Change vs preprocedure (%)	(+43.7)	(+21.8)	<.001
CCS I (%)	30.8	23.8	.03
Change vs preprocedure (%)	(+14.9)	(+0.9)	.01
CCS II (%)	12.2	28.5	.01
Change vs preprocedure (%)	(−43.6)	(−22.3)	<.01
CCS III–IV (%)	3.9	17.2	.01
Changes vs preprocedure (%)	(−24.4)	(−9.1)	.01

SAQ scores are expressed as mean (95% CI).
CCS represented as % of population.
Abbreviation: CCS, Canadian Cardiovascular Society.

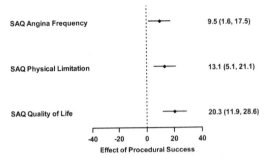

Fig. 8. Adjusted health status outcomes comparison between successful and unsuccessful PCI of CTO. Variables used in the model included age, gender, prior MI, hypertension, hyperlipidemia, diabetes, smoking status, prior CABG, number of diseased vessels, EF, preprocedure creatinine, β-blocker, calcium channel blocker and nitrate use, and hospital. Data are expressed as point estimate of change in outcome from baseline to follow-up with 95% CIs. (*From* Grantham JA, Jones PG, Cannon L, et al. Quantifying the early health status benefits of successful chronic total occlusion recanalization: results from the FlowCardia's Approach to Chronic Total Occlusion Recanalization (FACTOR) Trial. Circ Cardiovasc Qual Outcomes 2010; 3(3):284–90; with permission.)

and colleagues[25] looked at left ventriculography at baseline and at 6 months after successful treatment of 95 patients with CTO. LV function was assessed using LVEF and LV regional radial shortening. Using computer-assisted analysis, there was improvement in LVEF from 0.62 ± 0.13 at baseline to 0.67 ± 0.11 at follow-up ($P<.001$) after successful recanalization of the CTO. Regional radial shortening increased in the territory of the recanalized artery by 16% from 0.28 ± 0.11 to 0.32 ± 0.11 ($P<.001$). This increase was noted only in those patients whose artery was patent at follow-up and not significantly different in patients in whom the artery had reoccluded. In multiple regression analysis using angiographic and clinical data as independent variables, only baseline ejection fraction (EF) and occlusion of the treated artery were significantly related to change in the EF. The preprocedure angina class, duration of occlusion, and history of a prior MI were each nonstatistically significantly related to change in the EF after successful intervention.

Chung and colleagues[26] published a consecutive series of patients with angina or an abnormal exercise stress test that had treatment of a CTO. They divided the patients into 2 groups. Group 1 was composed of patients without a prior MI and group 2 was a well-matched group of patients with a prior MI. A subgroup of group 2 (with a prior MI) patients who had grade 3 collaterals had improvement in LV EF after CTO recanalization similar to those in group 1 (without a prior MI), implying that the collaterals in some way protected the viability of the myocardium that was presumed to be infarcted. Similarly, regional wall motion improved in the territories revascularized in group 1 but did not in group 2 (as shown in **Fig. 9**). Werner and colleagues[27] demonstrated that even though the presence of collaterals may influence the success of the interventional procedure, it did not predict the recovery of LV function. The LV function recovery depended on the integrity of the microcirculation, which is not visible by angiography.

Investigators at the Erasmus Medical Center studied the utility of CTO recanalization of dysfunctional yet viable segments of myocardium using preintervention and postintervention cardiac MRI study.[28] In their cohort of 27 patients, they found that the end-systolic and end-diastolic dimensions of the ventricle improved after successful recanalization of the occluded artery (**Fig. 10**). They also elegantly demonstrated that the extent of dysfunctional yet viable myocardium correlated with the improvement in the indices of end-systolic volumes/ejection fraction and systolic wall thickness (**Fig. 11**).

Investigators at Kings College London and the University of Toronto evaluated the preprocedure and postprocedure EF and transmural extent of infarction by MRI after recanalization of 30 CTO patients with drug-eluting stent.[29] Their conclusions were similar to those of prior studies, which showed improvement of global EF and segmental wall thickening in dysfunctional yet viable myocardium after CTO recanalization (**Fig. 12**). They also suggested that the transmural extent of infarction noted on preprocedure MRI can help predict the extent of expected improvement.

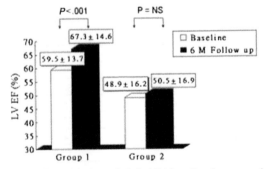

Fig. 9. The evolution of global LV function in groups 1 and 2 showing striking difference between the two groups. (*From* Chung CM, Nakamura S, Tanaka K, et al. Effect of recanalization of chronic total occlusions on global and regional left ventricular function in patients with or without previous myocardial infarction. Catheter Cardiovasc Interv 2003;60(3):368–74; with permission.)

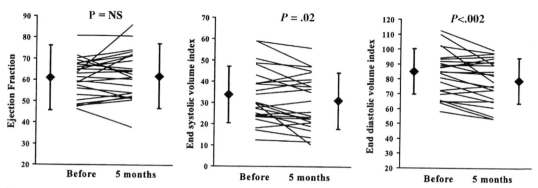

Fig. 10. The change in LV volume indexes between baseline and 5 months of follow-up measured with MRI. (*From* Baks T, van Geuns RJ, Duncker DJ, et al. Prediction of left ventricular function after drug-eluting stent implantation for chronic total coronary occlusions. J Am Coll Cardiol 2006;47(4):721–5; with permission.)

IMPROVEMENT IN ISCHEMIC BURDEN AFTER REVASCULARIZATION

Frequently, on diagnostic angiograms, large collaterals are noted to supply the territory of the CTO. This is often mentioned as a rationale for managing patients conservatively and deferring an intervention on CTO. This is a misconception based on the view that the collateral circulation is preventing the development of ischemia in the territory of the CTO.

Werner and colleagues[27] performed direct assessment of collateral function by measuring pressure and flow velocity in the collateralized epicardial segment distal to the occlusion. Doppler velocity was measured with the Doppler guide wire to record the average peak velocity as the area under the flow velocity curve before and after treatment of the CTO. The ratio of before-and-after

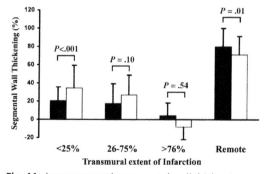

Fig. 11. Improvement in segmental wall thickening was related to the transmural extent of infarction assessed with MRI before revascularization. Solid bars before revascularization; open bars 5 months after revascularization. (*From* Baks T, van Geuns RJ, Duncker DJ, et al. Prediction of left ventricular function after drug-eluting stent implantation for chronic total coronary occlusions. J Am Coll Cardiol 2006;47(4):721–5; with permission.)

treatment flow velocities was used to arrive at the collateral flow index. For pressure recording, a pressure wire (Radi Medical System) was used to calculate the collateral pressure index (CPI). Adequate collateral supply has been previously defined and includes (1) distal pressure greater than 45 mm Hg and (2) CPI greater than 0.30. Thresholds for collateral function parameters insufficient to prevent ischemia were exceeded in 58% of patients using the distal pressure as the cutoff and when using CPI in 78% of patients.

The relationship between ischemia reduction and CTO recanalization has been studied by Safley and colleagues.[30] The aim of their study was to evaluate potential for reduction in ischemic burden, as assessed by myocardial perfusion imaging (MPI) after CTO PCI, and to attempt to establish thresholds associated with improvement of ischemia on follow-up MPI after CTO PCI. MPI studies included exercise or pharmacologic single-photon emission CT (SPECT) or PET imaging protocols. The results were stratified by their initial MPI summed difference score (SDS). The SDS was converted to a percentage of ischemic myocardium. Patients were stratified into 4 groups based on the SDS: SDS less than 4—normal/minimal ischemia (<5% of ischemic myocardium); SDS 4 to 8—mild ischemia (5%–9.9% of ischemic myocardium); SDS 9 to 13—moderate ischemia (10%–16% of ischemic myocardium); and SDS greater than 13—severe ischemia (>16%). A meaningful change in ischemic burden was defined as SDS greater than 4 corresponding with a 5% decrease in ischemic myocardium, which has been associated with decreased risk for death or MI (Clinical Outcomes Utilizing Revascularization and Aggressive Drug Evaluation [COURAGE] nuclear substudy[31]). In search of a threshold of ischemia that might be used to predict improvement, receiver

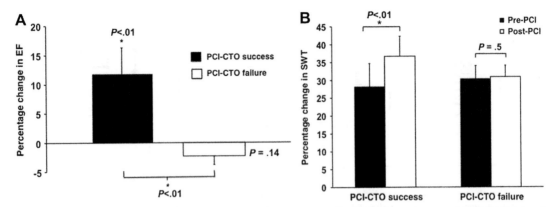

Fig. 12. (*A*) Effect of PCI of true CTO on global LV function and effect of PCI on segmental wall thickening in dysfunctional but viable segments. (*B*) Effect of PCI on segmental wall thickening in dysfunctional but viable segments. (*From* Paul GA, Connelly K, Zia Mo, et al. Impact of percutaneous coronary intervention of chronic total occlusion on left ventricular function using cardiac magnetic resonance imaging. J Cardiovasc Magn Reson 2011;13(Suppl 1):M6. © 2011 Paul et al; open access.)

operating characteristic (ROC) curves were generated. The Youden index[32] was used to define the optimal ischemic burden to predict improvement (**Figs. 13** and **14**). Not only does ischemic burden improve significantly in patients in whom baseline ischemia is moderate to high but also in the long term translates to a mortality benefit (**Fig. 15**).

The 4 important conclusions from this study were as follows: (1) mean reduction in ischemic burden after CTO PCI was 6.2% ± 6.0%; (2) a baseline LV ischemic burden of 12.5% was the optimal threshold predictive of improvement after CTO PCI; (3) a baseline LV ischemic burden of less than 6.25% was predictive of worsening ischemia after CTO PCI; and (4) if reduction in ischemic burden greater than 5% was achieved post PCI,

patients experienced fewer clinical events, in particular death and target vessel revascularization. This was the first attempt to establish objective criteria by which a rationale can be provided for CTO PCI. Using this information as a guide, an algorithm can be formulated for treatment of CTO based on MPI findings (**Fig. 16**).

One limitation of this study is that only 23% of all the CTOs attempted in the time frame were included in the study. There also exists a verification bias that might have an impact on the validity of the thresholds established by the ROC (**Fig. 17**). This was a single-center experience, which limits

Fig. 13. Changes in SDS by severity of baseline ischemia assessed by SPECT imaging 12 months before and after CTO PCI. (*From* Safley DM, Koshy S, Grantham JA, et al. Changes in myocardial ischemic burden following percutaneous coronary intervention of chronic total occlusions. Catheter Cardiovasc Interv 2011;78(3):337–43; with permission.)

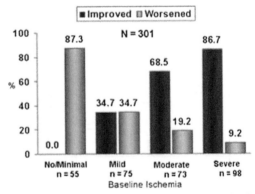

$P < .001$ for the trend of more improvement with greater ischemia at baseline

$P < .001$ for the trend of more decrease with less ischemia at baseline

Fig. 14. Percentage of patients with greater than 5% improvement in ischemic burden after CTO PCI stratified according to baseline ischemic burden. (*From* Safley DM, Koshy S, Grantham JA, et al. Changes in myocardial ischemic burden following percutaneous coronary intervention of chronic total occlusions. Catheter Cardiovasc Interv 2011;78(3):337–43; with permission.)

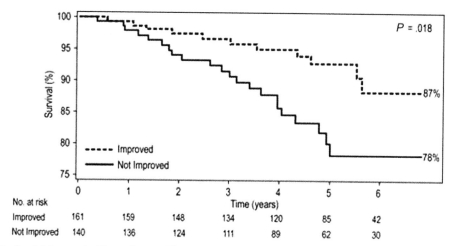

Fig. 15. Kaplan-Meier survival in patients with versus without improvement in ischemia on MPI. (*From* Safley DM, Koshy S, Grantham JA, et al. Changes in myocardial ischemic burden following percutaneous coronary intervention of chronic total occlusions. Catheter Cardiovasc Interv 2011;78(3):337–43; with permission.)

the applicability of the findings to the general population, especially when this single center achieved a 98% success rate in treating these complex lesions. This experience, however, lays the foundation for further investigation in this area of ischemia-guided CTO PCI.

Improved Tolerance for Future Ischemic Events

CTO is considered the hallmark of an endured MI that has not been treated with reperfusion.[33] A previous MI is a known predictor for impaired clinical outcome irrespective of reduced LV function.[34] Presence of a CTO may, therefore, identify a subset of patients with a poor clinical outcome in the setting of ST elevation myocardial infarction (STEMI).

Recent studies have shown that patients with a CTO in non-IRAs are a subgroup of patients with multivessel disease (MVD) who are truly at risk after primary PCI is performed for STEMI.[35,36] In this setting, van der Schaaf and colleagues[36] were the first to demonstrate a higher 1-year mortality rate in patients with MVD and the presence of a CTO in a non-IRA. After adjustment for possible confounders by multivariate Cox regression analysis, MVD without CTO was not predictive of mortality. Similar results were reported by this group in a cohort consisting exclusively of STEMI patients with cardiogenic shock.[37] The landmark survival analysis at 5-year follow-up showed that CTO in a non-IRA was a strong independent predictor of 30-day, 1-year, and 5-year mortality. MVD without a CTO was only a weak predictor of 30-day mortality and not an independent predictor

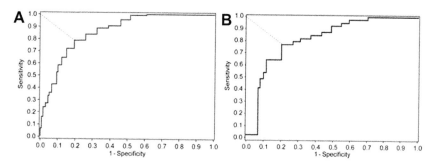

Fig. 16. ROC curves predicting decreases (*A*) and increases (*B*) in ischemia greater than or equal to 5% after CTO PCI. (*A*) ROC analysis identified a 12.5% ischemic burden as the optimal cutpoint to predict improvement in ischemia after CTO PCI (sensitivity 80%, specificity 80%). (*B*) ROC curve analysis identified 6.25% ischemic burden as the optimal cutpoint to predict worsening in ischemia after CTO PCI (sensitivity 75%, specificity 80%). (*From* Safley DM, Koshy S, Grantham JA, et al. Changes in myocardial ischemic burden following percutaneous coronary intervention of chronic total occlusions. Catheter Cardiovasc Interv 2011;78(3):337–43; with permission.)

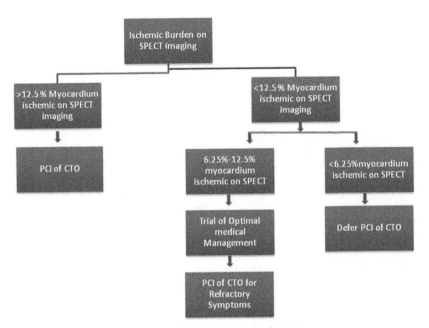

Fig. 17. Proposed treatment algorithm for CTO based on ischemia by MPI.

of 1-year and 5-year mortality. Furthermore, CTO, and not MVD alone, is associated with both a reduced LVEF after the index event and a further deterioration in LVEF within the first year thereafter.[38,39]

A study by Lexis and colleagues[33] extended the data available from the Thrombus Aspiration during Percutaneous Coronary Intervention in Acute Myocardial Infarction Study (TAPAS) to provide a mechanistic substrate for observations made in the aforementioned studies. Their study showed that patients with CTO in a non-IRAs demonstrated a lower myocardial blush grade, decreased ST segment resolution, and increased persistence of ST-segment deviation There was also a significantly larger enzymatic infarction size in patients with STEMI and a concomitant CTO compared with patients without a CTO. Furthermore, the presence of a CTO in non-IRAs in STEMI patients was a risk factor for cardiac mortality, all-cause mortality, and MACE. These observations imply that the unfavorable outcome and poor tolerance to an ischemic event (STEMI) observed in this study can be explained in part by the more severely impaired myocardial perfusion and larger enzymatic infarct size in patients with concomitant CTOs. It is conceivable that patients with CTO have a lower potential for collateral blood supply to the infarcted area because they only have 1 of 2 possible remaining coronary arteries at their disposal for collateral blood to supply the IRA. Conversely, an abrupt reduction in collateral flow from the IRA to the CTO-related

myocardium may lead to additional myocardial necrosis.[33,40] Other factors that might contribute to the poor tolerance of STEMI with concomitant CTOs include the lack of a compensation mechanism for the decrease in the LVEF after acute MI and a greater risk profile in those patients with CTO (diabetes, previous MI, lower LVEF, lower baseline TIMI scores, and cardiogenic shock on admission).[39]

Although the presence of a CTO is an ominous sign in STEMI patients, the clinical benefit of CTO recanalization during the index hospitalization is currently unknown. Potentially, opening a CTO can (1) restore contractile function of a hibernated myocardium and (2) improve perfusion at overlapping regions at the infarct border zone. This could improve healing in the border zone, protect against negative remodeling, and possibly translate to a more preserved residual LV function and improved survival. A study by Yang and colleagues[41] was the first to report that successful staged revascularization of a CTO in a non-IRA is associated with improved survival and reduced MACE in patients with acute STEMI treated with primary PCI. This study had several limitations. This was a single-center observational study with a small sample size. The follow-up was only 2 years and it is not known if the beneficial effects persist over time. Finally, detailed ischemic status of the CTO territory in asymptomatic patients before staged revascularization was lacking. The ongoing Evaluating XIENCE V and Left Ventricular Function in Percutaneous Coronary Intervention on Occlusions after ST-Elevation

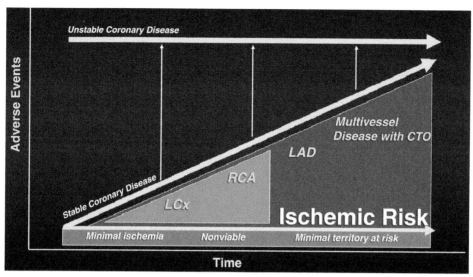

Fig. 18. Ischemic risk model for coronary disease with predictable/stable symptoms: a decision matrix for CTO revascularization current outcomes data suggests that adverse events for coronary disease can be risk predicted by coronary disease burden (eg, phenotyped multivessel coronary disease) and magnitude and degree of ischemia. In this revascularization decision matrix model, coronary disease is not assumed to be intrinsically stable on the basis of predictable symptoms but rather as a risk continuum. In this model, patients at higher risk are more likely to destabilize and transition to acute syndromes, MI, and death. The highest-risk patients seem to have the greatest magnitude of benefit from revascularization. Benefits from revascularization are presumed to be greatest for patients with multivessel disease with CTO and left anterior descending coronary artery (LAD) CTO, followed by single-vessel RCA or left circumflex artery (LCx) CTO with high ischemic burden. This risk continuum might represent a framework to substratify (in addition to symptomatic status) and determine revascularization, including that for CTO, for patients with nonacute coronary artery disease. (*From* Thompson CA. Percutaneous revascularization of coronary chronic total occlusions: the new era begins. JACC Cardiovasc Interv 2010;3(2):152–4; with permission.)

Myocardial Infarction (EXPLORE) trial is the first randomized, prospective, multicenter, 2-arm trial with blinded endpoints and 5-year clinical follow-up that is powered to investigate whether staged recanalization of a CTO in a non-IRA after primary PCI for STEMI results in a better preserved residual LVEF, reduced end-diastolic volume, and enhanced clinical outcome using cardiac MRI.[42] The results of this trial should help evolve a strategy for CTO revascularization in non-IRAs after primary PCI for STEMI.

SUMMARY

In summary, the field of CTO PCI is a rapidly expanding and exciting area of research. The observational studies (described previously) show a trend toward clinical benefits in carefully selected groups of patients with symptoms or ischemic risk burden as described in the decision matrix for CTO revascularization (**Fig. 18**). With contemporary strategies and techniques, the success rate in experienced operators can exceed 90%. This will hopefully open the door for performance of randomized controlled trials comparing CTO PCI with optimal medical management in patients with stable coronary artery disease.

REFERENCES

1. Stone GS, Kandzari DE, Mehran R, et al. Percutaneous recanalization of chronic totally occluded arteries: a consensus document. Part I. Circulation 2005;112:2364–72.
2. Christofferson RD, Lehmann KG, Martin GV, et al. Effect of chronic total coronary occlusion on treatment strategy. Am J Cardiol 2005;95:1088–91.
3. Grantham JA, Marso SP, Spertus J, et al. Chronic total occlusion angioplasty in the United States. JACC Cardiovasc Interv 2009;2:479–86.
4. Hochman JS, Lamas GA, Buller CE, et al. Coronary intervention for persistent occlusion after myocardial infarction. N Engl J Med 2006;355(23): 2395–407.
5. Srivatsa SS, Edwards WD, Boos CM, et al. Histologic correlates of angiographic chronic total coronary artery occlusions influence of occlusion duration on neovascular channel patterns and intimal plaque composition. J Am Coll Cardiol 1997; 29:955–63.

6. Katsuragawa M, Fujiwara H, Miyamae M, et al. Histologic studies in percutaneous transluminal coronary angioplasty for chronic total occlusion: comparison of tapering and abrupt types of occlusion and short and long occluded segments. J Am Coll Cardiol 1993;21:604–11.

7. Finn AV, Kolodgie FD, Nakano M, et al. The differences between neovascularization of chronic total occlusion and intraplaque angiogenesis. JACC Cardiovasc Imaging 2010;3(8):806–10.

8. Suero JA, Marso SP, Jones PG, et al. Procedural outcomes and long term survival among patients undergoing percutaneous coronary intervention of a chronic total occlusion in native coronary arteries: a 20 year experience. J Am Coll Cardiol 2001;38(2):409–14.

9. Olivari Z, Rubartelli P, Piscione F, et al. Immediate results and one year clinical outcomes after percutaneous coronary interventions in chronic total occlusions. J Am Coll Cardiol 2003;41:1672–8.

10. Hoye A, van Domburg RT, Sonnenschein K, et al. Percutaneous coronary intervention for chronic total occlusions: the thoraxcenter experience. 1992-2002. Eur Heart J 2005;26:2630–6.

11. Prasad A, Rihal CS, Lennon RJ, et al. Trends in outcomes after percutaneous coronary intervention for chronic total occlusions: a 25 year experience from the Mayo Clinic. J Am Coll Cardiol 2007;49:1611–8.

12. Aziz S, Stables RH, Grayson AD, et al. Percutaneous coronary intervention for chronic total occlusions: improved survival for patients with successful procedure compared to a failed procedure. Catheter Cardiovasc Interv 2007;70:15–20.

13. Valenti R, Migliorini A, Signorini U, et al. Impact of complete revascularization with percutaneous coronary intervention on survival in patients with at least one chronic total occlusion. Eur Heart J 2008;29(19):2336–42.

14. Safley DA, House JA, Marso SP, et al. Improvement in survival following percutaneous coronary intervention of coronary chronic total occlusions: variability by target vessel. JACC Cardiovasc Interv 2008;1:295–302.

15. Lee SW, Lee JY, Park DW, et al. Long term clinical outcomes of successful versus unsuccessful revascularization with drug eluting stents for true chronic total occlusions. Catheter Cardiovasc Interv 2011;78:346–53.

16. de Labriolle A, Bonello L, Roy P, et al. Comparison of safety, efficacy, and outcome of successful versus unsuccessful percutaneous coronary intervention in "true" chronic total occlusions. Am J Cardiol 2008;102:1175–81.

17. Joyal D, Afilalo J, Rinfret S. Effectiveness of recanalization of chronic total occlusions: a systematic review and meta-analysis. Am Heart J 2010;160(1):179–87.

18. Werner GS, Gitt AK, Zeymer U, et al. Chronic total coronary occlusions in patients with stable angina pectoris: impact on therapy and outcome in present day clinical practice. Clin Res Cardiol 2009;98(7):435–41.

19. Ruocco NA Jr, Ring ME, Holubkov R, et al. Results of coronary angioplasty of chronic total occlusions (the National Heart, Lung, and Blood Institute 1985-1986 Percutaneous Transluminal Angioplasty Registry). Am J Cardiol 1992;69(1):69–76.

20. Bell MR, Berger PB, Bresnahan JF, et al. Initial and long-term outcome of 354 patients after coronary balloon angioplasty of total coronary artery occlusions. Circulation 1992;85(3):1003–11.

21. Noguchi T, Miyazaki S, Morii I, et al. Percutaneous transluminal coronary angioplasty of chronic total occlusions. Determinants of primary success and long-term clinical outcome. Catheter Cardiovasc Interv 2000;49(3):258–64.

22. Garratt AM, Hutchinson A, Russell I, et al. The UK version of the Seattle Angina Questionnaire (SAQ-UK): reliability, validity and responsiveness. J Clin Epidemiol 2001;54(9):907–15.

23. Borgia F, Viceconte N, Ali O, et al. Improved cardiac survival, freedom from mace and angina-related quality of life after successful percutaneous recanalization of coronary artery chronic total occlusions. Int J Cardiol 2011. [Epub ahead of print].

24. Grantham JA, Jones PG, Cannon L, et al. Quantifying the early health status benefits of successful chronic total occlusion recanalization: results from the FlowCardia's Approach to Chronic Total Occlusion Recanalization (FACTOR) Trial. Circ Cardiovasc Qual Outcomes 2010;3(3):284–90.

25. Sirnes PA, Myreng Y, Mølstad P, et al. Improvement in left ventricular ejection fraction and wall motion after successful recanalization of chronic coronary occlusions. Eur Heart J 1998;19(2):273–81.

26. Chung CM, Nakamura S, Tanaka K, et al. Effect of recanalization of chronic total occlusions on global and regional left ventricular function in patients with or without previous myocardial infarction. Catheter Cardiovasc Interv 2003;60(3):368–74.

27. Werner GS, Surber R, Ferrari M, et al. The functional reserve of collaterals supplying long-term chronic total coronary occlusions in patients without prior myocardial infarction. Eur Heart J 2006;27(20):2406–12.

28. Baks T, van Geuns RJ, Duncker DJ, et al. Prediction of left ventricular function after drug-eluting stent implantation for chronic total coronary occlusions. J Am Coll Cardiol 2006;47(4):721–5.

29. Paul GA, Connelly K, Zia Mo, et al. Impact of percutaneous coronary intervention of chronic total occlusion on left ventricular function using cardiac magnetic resonance imaging. J Cardiovasc Magn Reson 2011;13(Suppl 1):M6.

30. Safley DM, Koshy S, Grantham JA, et al. Changes in myocardial ischemic burden following percutaneous coronary intervention of chronic total occlusions. Catheter Cardiovasc Interv 2011;78(3):337–43.

31. Shaw LJ, Berman DS, Maron DJ, et al. Optimal medical therapy with or without percutaneous coronary intervention to reduce ischemic burden: results from the Clinical Outcomes Utilizing Revascularization and Aggressive Drug Evaluation (COURAGE) trial nuclear substudy. Circulation 2008;117(10):1283–91.

32. Perkins NJ, Schisterman EF. The Youden Index and the optimal cut-point corrected for measurement error. Biom J 2005;47(4):428–41.

33. Lexis CP, van der Horst IC, Rahel BM, et al. Impact of chronic total occlusions on markers of reperfusion, infarct size, and long-term mortality: a substudy from the tapas-trial. Catheter Cardiovasc Interv 2011;77:484–91.

34. Acampa W, Petretta M, Spinelli L, et al. Survival benefit after revascularization is independent of left ventricular ejection fraction improvement in patients with previous myocardial infarction and viable myocardium. Eur J Nucl Med Mol Imaging 2005;32:430–7.

35. Moreno R, Conde C, Perez-Vizcayno MJ, et al. Prognostic impact of a chronic occlusion in a noninfarct vessel in patients with acute myocardial infarction and multivessel disease undergoing primary percutaneous coronary intervention. J Invasive Cardiol 2006;18:16–9.

36. van der Schaaf RJ, Vis MM, Sjauw KD, et al. Impact of multivessel coronary disease on long-term mortality in patients with st-elevation myocardial infarction is due to the presence of a chronic total occlusion. Am J Cardiol 2006;98:1165–9.

37. van der Schaaf RJ, Claessen BE, Vis MM, et al. Effect of multivessel coronary disease with or without concurrent chronic total occlusion on one-year mortality in patients treated with primary percutaneous coronary intervention for cardiogenic shock. Am J Cardiol 2010;105:955–9.

38. Claessen BE, van der Schaaf RJ, Verouden NJ, et al. Evaluation of the effect of a concurrent chronic total occlusion on long-term mortality and left ventricular function in patients after primary percutaneous coronary intervention. JACC Cardiovasc Interv 2009;2: 1128–34.

39. Tajstra M, Gasior M, Gierlotka M, et al. Comparison of five-year outcomes of patients with and without chronic total occlusion of noninfarct coronary artery after primary coronary intervention for ST-segment elevation acute myocardial infarction. Am J Cardiol 2012;109(2):208–13.

40. Belardi JA. 1 is manageable but 2 may be 2 much: shall we open ctos? Catheter Cardiovasc Interv 2011;77:492–3.

41. Yang ZK, Zhang RY, Hu J, et al. Impact of successful staged revascularization of a chronic total occlusion in the non-infarct-related artery on long-term outcome in patients with acute st-segment elevation myocardial infarction. Int J Cardiol 2011. [Epub ahead of print].

42. van der Schaaf RJ, Claessen BE, Hoebers LP, et al, Investigators Explore. Rationale and design of explore: a randomized, prospective, multicenter trial investigating the impact of recanalization of a CTO on left ventricular function in patients after primary percutaneous coronary intervention for acute st-elevation myocardial infarction. Trials 2010;11:89.

Toolbox and Inventory Requirements for Chronic Total Occlusion Percutaneous Coronary Interventions

Khaldoon Alaswad, MD, RVT

KEYWORDS

- Coronary • Chronic • Occlusion • Intervention • Equipment

KEY POINTS

- The toolbox and inventory requirements to establish a successful chronic total occlusion (CTO) percutaneous coronary intervention (PCI) program are limited and not expensive.
- Two arterial accesses are needed in most CTO PCI procedures using radial and common femoral arteries. Large-bore 7F to 8F and long 45 to 55 cm sheaths are used in the common femoral artery, whereas the radial artery cannot tolerate sheaths larger than 6F or longer than 11 cm. Supportive guide catheters are needed for CTO PCI, enhancement of the guide catheter support is frequently needed during CTO PCI.
- Limited coronary guide wires types are needed to perform most CTO PCI techniques. Small bend at the tip of the wire is the most common wire shaping for CTO PCI.
- Innovative techniques, such as dissection and reentry, and retrograde approaches are performed as primary revascularization strategies with the advent of equipment such as the Bridgepoint system (BridgePoint Medical, Inc., Plymouth, MN, USA).
- Complications management equipment is an important part of the CTO PCI toolbox, to treat perforations and vessel ruptures with coils and stent grafts.

The recanalization of a coronary chronic total occlusion (CTO), defined as an occlusion in a coronary artery with thrombolysis in myocardial infarction 0 flow for at least 3 months, is the latest frontier in percutaneous coronary intervention (PCI).[1] The perceived increased cost, the lack of a well-defined approach to CTO PCI, and the relatively low success rate (50%–70%) have made interventional cardiologists reluctant to attempt CTO PCI (attempt rates 11.7% and 13.6% during 2004–2007).[2] The finding of a coronary CTO is one of the most common reasons for referral to coronary artery bypass grafting surgery (CABG).[3] Patient referral to CABG does not guarantee revascularization of the artery with a CTO; the Synergy Between PCI with Taxus and Cardiac Surgery (SYNTAX) clinical trial, showed that chronically occluded coronary arteries were frequently left untreated even during CABG, only 69% of the CTO segments received bypass grafting and complete revascularization was achieved in 49.6%.[4–6] On other hand, CTO PCI success rates above 85% have been achieved.[2]

The Japanese CTO PCI operators have pioneered several CTO PCI techniques and equipment.[7,8] More recently, a group of North American interventional cardiologists formed the North American Total Occlusion group (the NATO group). The NATO group established a new school in CTO PCI, more in tune with the economic and regulatory environment in North America.[2,9] The NATO group focuses on expanding the CTO PCI

Appleton Heart Institute, 1818 North Meade Street, Appleton, WI 54911, USA
E-mail address: kalaswad@gmail.com

Intervent Cardiol Clin 1 (2012) 281–297
doi:10.1016/j.iccl.2012.03.002
2211-7458/12/$ – see front matter © 2012 Elsevier Inc. All rights reserved.

interventional.theclinics.com

outside highly specialized centers by developing algorithms that simplify the decision-making tree and equipment choices. The NATO group emphasizes the importance of quickly and safely moving the gear (coronary guide wire and microcatheter) to a position (base of operation) that facilitates entry or reentry into the artery true lumen beyond the occluded segment.

Although the general principles are the same, CTO PCI is different than non–CTO PCI in several aspects (**Table 1**). CTO PCI operators need to acquire additional skills, including collateral crossing and dissection and reentry techniques.[6,9,10] Additional guide catheter support is frequently needed during equipment introduction and base of operation changes. Despite the differences between CTO PCI and non–CTO PCI, few additional devices are needed when embarking on a successful CTO PCI program development (see **Table 1**).

This article focuses on the equipment necessary to develop a successful CTO PCI program. The equipment discussion in this article follows the steps of the CTO PCI procedure to discuss necessary arterial access equipment, guide catheters, CTO PCI coronary guide wires, microcatheters, dissection and reentry equipment, and other specialized equipment used during the CTO PCI procedure.

ARTERIAL ACCESS EQUIPMENT

Contralateral coronary angiography alone or simultaneous with ipsilateral coronary angiography is important during CTO PCI, even if the retrograde technique was not used during the recanalization procedure. Two arterial accesses should be established in most CTO PCI procedures.[2] Bilateral common femoral artery (CFA) accesses are most commonly used; few operators use bilateral radial artery (RA) accesses, whereas others use a hybrid approach by combining a CFA access with an access from a radial artery.

The preferred sheath from the CFA is a large bore (7–8F, 45–55 cm long). Long large-bore sheaths provide more room for equipment and better tactile feedback and wire manipulation. More access site complications are obvious disadvantages of the larger sheaths when compared with 6F sheaths.[11]

The sheaths for the RA access are mostly 6F in diameter and 11 cm long. Longer sheaths in the RA might increase the risk of spasm and sheath entrapment. Few patients can tolerate sheaths larger than 6F in the RA. The sheathless guide catheters from the RA provide a 7.5F lumen in a 5F arterial puncture; however, these sheathless guide catheters are not widely available in the United States and it is difficult to stabilize these highly slippery guide catheters in the coronary artery ostium. Advantages of the RA access are less bleeding, fewer vascular complications, less pain, improved quality of life, and early ambulation.[11,12] Less guide catheter support and less room for devices are obvious disadvantages of 6F guide catheters from the RA access. Another important disadvantage of a 6F guide catheter in a CTO PCI procedure is the inability to deliver a stent graft, which needs at least a 7F guide catheter. Interventional cardiologists who use the RA access must use the ping-pong guide catheters technique,[13] in case of a coronary artery rupture, in which another guide catheter is advanced to the same coronary artery ostium from a different arterial access. The CFA access is used in case of an iatrogenic coronary artery rupture to accommodate the large bore sheath and guide catheter necessary for the bulky equipment used in perforation control.

GUIDE CATHETERS

The ideal CTO PCI guide catheter should provide coaxial engagement, good back-up support, large

Table 1
Equipment and procedural differences between CTO PCI and non–CTO PCI

	CTO PCI	Non–CTO PCI
Arterial access sheaths	7–8F, 45 cm long in the CFA 6–7F, 11 cm long in the RA	6F 11 cm
Guide catheters	7–8F 90 cm from the CFA 6–7F 90 cm in the RA	5–6F regular length
Coronary angiography	Bilateral coronary angiography	Ipsilateral coronary angiography only
Coronary guide wire	Specially designed wires	Regular work-horse wires
Guide wire support	Microcatheter support usually required	Microcatheter support rarely required

Abbreviations: CFA, common femoral artery; RA, radial artery.

lumen to accommodate multiple devices simultaneously, enough range for wire externalization, and a nontraumatic tip (**Table 2**).

The guide catheter engaged in the occluded coronary artery or the left main coronary artery (LMCA), if the occlusion is in the left anterior descending coronary artery or the left circumflex coronary artery, is called the antegrade guide catheter, whereas the guide catheter engaged in the contralateral coronary artery to the occluded artery is called the retrograde guide catheter. Wire externalization might not be achievable with the usual 100 cm long guide catheters and the available 300 cm long coronary guide wires, especially when using a microcatheter with the coronary guide wire. Manufacturers make 80, 85, and 90 cm long guide catheters to facilitate wire externalization. There are two techniques to shorten the guide catheter if premade 90 cm or shorter guide catheters are not available. Operators can cut a 10 cm to 15 cm long piece of the guide catheter and use a segment of 1F smaller than the guide catheter sheath to recreate the guide catheter[10] or cut the proximal hub and use a Ureteral Catheter Connecter (Cook Urological, Spencer, IN, USA) as a hub for guide catheter.

Side holes close to the distal end of the guide catheter are frequently necessary during CTO PCI procedures, especially when using a large bore guide catheter to engage the right coronary artery (RCA). Although the side holes allow perfusion during a snug engagement of the coronary artery ostium, they do not prevent guide catheter injury to the ostium.

In cases where the ipsilateral coronary collaterals must be used for coronary guide wire externalization, the operator should use an 8F guide catheter to accommodate the retrograde and antegrade equipment in the same catheter, or a ping-pong guide catheters technique.

Owing to anatomic orientation, a guide catheter from the right RA access usually provides better support in the left coronary artery, whereas a guide catheter from the left RA access provides better support in the RCA.

CORONARY GUIDE WIRES FOR CTO PCI

Mastering the skills of coronary guide wire manipulation and gaining the experience of tactile feedback are important operator skills for CTO PCI. Crossing a CTO is different than passing a guide wire through a stenosis while a channel is seen by angiography. Inability to cross the occluded coronary segment with the guide wire is the most common mode of failure in the CTO PCI[1]; in addition, CTO PCI coronary guide wires induce perforations more frequently than spring tip coronary guide wires used in non–CTO PCI. Limiting the wire selections during the CTO PCI facilitates mastering the wire techniques and increases procedure efficiency. Multiple coronary guide wires with different characteristics are frequently needed to achieve various functions during the CTO PCI procedure (**Box 1**).

Wire shaping in the CTO PCI is different than the non–CTO PCI (**Fig. 1**). The 30° to 45° bend at the last 1 mm from the wire tip of the coronary guide wire facilitates microchannel finding and cap penetration, and avoids side branches and unintended dissections. To reenter the true lumen from the subintimal space, the wire tip bind should be more acute and the bent segment should be longer (see **Fig. 1**). To perform subintimal dissection the wire tip is shaped in a knuckle-like "umbrella handle" 2 to 3 mm from the distal end (see **Fig. 1**).

Table 2
The most commonly used guide catheters during CTO PCI[a]

Left Coronary Artery	Right Coronary Artery
EBU 3.75, 4, 4.5 (Medtronic, Minneapolis, MN, USA)	Judkins Right 4
XB 3.5, 4, 4.5 (Cordis Corporation Warren/Bridgewater, NJ, USA)	Amplatz 0.75, 1
Voda Left and CLS Curve (Boston Scientific, Natick, MA, USA)	Hockey stick

[a] Other guide catheter shapes that provide passive support can be used.

Box 1
Guide wire functions in the CTO PCI
Microchannels probing and crossing
Collateral circulation crossing for retrograde CTO PCI techniques
Proximal or distal occlusion cap penetration
Knuckle dissection
Reentry into the true coronary artery lumen after dissection

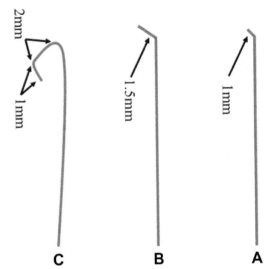

Fig. 1. Coronary guide wire shapes for CTO PCI. (*A*) Wire shape to penetrate the occlusion cap or to find a microchannel. (*B*) Wire shape to reenter into the true lumen from the subintimal space. (*C*) Wire shape for controlled subintimal dissection.

FUNCTIONAL CTO CORONARY GUIDE WIRES CLASSIFICATION

The CTO PCI coronary guide wires can be divided functionally in two major categories at the current stage of wire technology (**Fig. 2**): polymer-jacketed wires (hydrophilic) that provide less tactile feedback and non–polymer-jacketed (non-hydrophilic) wires that provide good tactile feed back during manipulation in the occluded coronary artery.

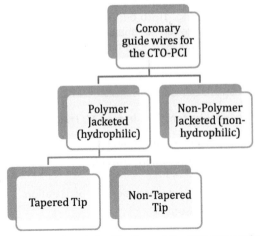

Fig. 2. Functional classification of the CTO PCI guide wires.

In addition to the work-horse coronary guide wires, only four essential wires are needed in catheterization laboratories embarking on developing a successful CTO PCI program. Other CTO schools, advocating gradual nonjacketed wire escalation, require a larger number of wires with different characteristics, such as the ASAHI MiracleBros coronary guide wires family (Abbott Laboratories, Abbott Park, IL, USA). Wire externalization during retrograde CTO PCI techniques frequently requires longer wires than the usual 300 cm wires commonly available in the catheterization laboratories (**Box 2**).

HOW TO CHOOSE A WIRE

There are several algorithms for wire selection during CTO PCI. The NATO group provides a simplified algorithm for wire choices (**Fig. 3**). The CTO features, the approach chosen, and the operator experience determine the CTO PCI coronary guide wire choice. Tapered polymer-jacketed wires with soft tips are made for a microchannel crossing even if the channel is not visible by angiography. Low tip-load polymer-jacketed wires can avoid unintended dissections in a tortuous calcified CTO. Stiff nonjacketed wires with good torque control are used to puncture the occlusion cap. These stiff wires should not be advanced beyond the occlusion cap if the course of the occluded segment is ambiguous. Dissection and reentry technique requires a polymer-jacketed wire to perform knuckle dissection, and a nonjacketed stiff wire with a specially bent tip for reentry into the true lumen from the subintimal space (see **Fig. 1**).

The following wires are most frequently used by the NATO group. These wire choices could change because of new designs and technologies (**Table 3**).

Fielder XT

The Fielder XT coronary guide wire (Abbott Laboratories, Abbott Park, IL, USA) is a polymer-jacketed wire that tapers to 0.009 in to facilitate

---

Box 2
Available 0.014 guide wires in North America for wire exteriorization during CTO PCI with a retrograde technique

ViperWire Advance Guide Wire, a 335 cm long (Cardiovascular Systems Inc, St Paul, MN, USA).

Rota Wire, 325 cm long (Boston Scientific, Natick, MA, USA).

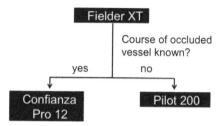

Fig. 3. Coronary guide wire selection algorithm in CTO PCI in the antegrade approach or after crossing the collateral in the retrograde approach. Fielder XT, Pilot 200, and Confianza Pro 12 guide wires (Abbott Laboratories, Abbott Park, IL, USA). (*Courtesy of* Dr William Lombardi.)

microchannel finding and crossing (see **Table 3**). When used to perform controlled dissection, the Fielder XT wire forms a small knuckle, which induces a small subintimal dissection space that facilitates reentry into the true lumen. This wire is used occasionally for collateral wire crossing, when there is a significant tortuosity.

Fielder FC

The Fielder FC coronary guide wire (Abbott Laboratories, Abbott Park, IL, USA) is a polymer-jacketed wire with a nontapered low-load tip to prevent dissections and perforations, especially during collateral channels crossing (see **Table 3**). Wire manipulation to cross the collateral circulation requires only torquing the wire with a bidirectional rotational movement without forward advancement; the wire should cross under its own weight.[10] Premature ventricular beats should alert the operators that the wire is not in the right channel.

Pilot 200

The Pilot 200 coronary guide wire (Abbott Laboratories, Abbott Park, IL, USA) is a polymer-jacketed wire with a high tip-load used to puncture a cap or

a dissection flap in order to enter or reenter the true lumen of an occluded coronary artery (see **Table 3**). This wire provides good pushability during knuckle dissection; however, the dissecting loop tends to become wider than the vessel outline.

Pilot 50

The Pilot 50 coronary guide wire (Abbott Laboratories, Abbott Park, IL, USA) is a polymer-jacketed wire with a nontapered low-load tip that functions like the Fielder FC but is less versatile in crossing the collateral channels. The Pilot 50 wire is frequently used in the wire swap technique (see later discussion).

Confianza Pro 12

The Confianza Pro 12 coronary guide wire (Abbott Laboratories, Abbott Park, IL, USA) is a non–polymer jacketed at the tip and provides excellent penetration and torquing abilities. Owing to its stiff and tapered tip (0.009 in), the Confianza Pro 12 coronary guide wire plays a major rule in cap penetration and true lumen reentry (see **Table 3**); however, anatomic ambiguity increases the risk of perforation and unintentional dissections. Operators use the Confianza Pro 12 coronary guide wire to puncture the proximal or the distal cap without farther wire advancement and then a polymer-jacketed wire is used to negotiate the rest of the occlusion.

MICROCATHETERS

Microcatheters are small-diameter catheters used to facilitate wire exchanges, keep wire position between wire exchanges, improve wire torque response, and provide backup support to the coronary guide wire. The ideal microcatheter in CTO PCI should have a low crossing profile to track into the occlusion, good pushability, and

Table 3
Commonly used coronary guide wires for coronary CTO PCI with specifications and functions

	Fielder XT	Fielder FC	Pilot 200	Confianza Pro 12
Coating	Polymer jacket	Polymer jacket	Polymer jacket	Hybrid coating
Tip load	1.2 g	1.6 g	4.1 g	12.4 g
Tip diameter	0.009 in	0.014 in	0.014 in	0.009 in
Functions	Finding and crossing microchannels Dissection	Collateral crossing True lumen finding after dissection	Cap penetration Lumen reentry Dissection	Cap penetration Lumen reentry

a small shaft diameter to share the space in the guide catheter with other equipment if needed.

The microcatheters provide dynamic wire tip load according to the distance of the wire tip protrusion from the end of the microcatheter. A 12 g wire tip load can be increased to 45 g with short protrusion of the wire outside the distal tip of the microcatheter (**Fig. 4**).[14]

The manufacturers add a radiopaque band to the distal tip to facilitate radiographic visibility and control of the coronary guide wire. Microcatheter distal tip visibility under fluoroscope is important, especially when negotiating a tortuous coronary vessel.

Multiple microcatheter brands are available for use in CTO PCI procedures (**Table 4**), but several CTO PCI operators use over-the-wire (OTW) 1.5 mm or smaller coronary angioplasty balloons as microcatheters. There are microcatheters designed for special functions in the CTO PCI procedures, such as the Corsair microcatheter (Asahi Intecc, Santa Ana, CA, USA) for collateral circulation crossing, the Venture wire control catheter (St Jude Medical, St Paul, MN, USA) or SuperCross microcatheter (Vascular Solutions, Inc, Minneapolis, MN, USA) for angulated coronary guide wire control, and the Tornus microcatheter (Asahi

Intecc, Santa Ana, CA, USA) for crossing calcified lesions over a coronary guide wire.

FineCross Microcatheter (Work-Hours Microcatheter)

The FineCross microcatheter (Terumo Medical Corporation, Somerset, NJ, USA) is available in two lengths, 135 cm and 150 cm. This microcatheter provides a small distal crossing profile (1.8F) and a very distal marker (**Fig. 5**). The FineCross microcatheter provides less pushability and wire support than the OTW coronary angioplasty balloon.

OTW Coronary Angioplasty Balloon as a Microcatheter

Several CTO PCI operators use a 1.5 mm or smaller OTW coronary angioplasty balloon instead of a more expensive microcatheter. OTW coronary angioplasty balloons provide good support to push the coronary guide wire through a stenosis or an occlusion, but less ability to track in a tortuous coronary segment. It is important to avoid coronary angioplasty balloons with two marker bands, because the distal marker band in most coronary angioplasty balloons increases

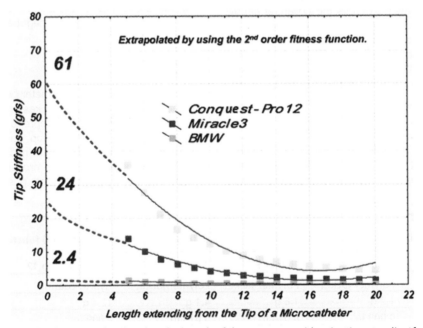

Fig. 4. The wire tip-load is inversely related to the length of the coronary guide wire tip extending from the tip of a microcatheter. BMW, Balance Middle Weight Coronary Guide wire (Abbott Laboratories, Abbott Park, IL, USA), Conqeust—Pro 12 coronary guide wire is equivalent to Confianza Pro 12 coronary guide wire (Abbott Laboratories. Abbott Park, IL, USA). Miracle 3 is a member of the Miracle coronary guide wire series (Abbott Laboratories. Abbott Park, IL, USA). (*From* Saito S. Wire control handling technique. In: Waksman R, Saito S, editors. Chronic total occlusions: a guide to recanalization. Hoboken (NJ): Wiley/Blackwell; 2009; with permission.)

Table 4
Currently available microcatheters

Manufacturer	Microcatheter	Length	Distal Diameter
Asahi	Corsair	135 cm, 150 cm	2.6F
	Tornus	150 cm	2.1 and 2.6F
Boston Scientific	Renegade	105 cm, 115 cm, 135 cm	2.8F
	Tracker Excel 14	150 cm	1.9F
	Excelsior 1018	150 cm	2.0F
Cordis	Transit	135 cm	2.5F
	Prowler	150 cm	1.9F
Spectranetics (The Spectranetics Corporation, Colorado Springs, CO, USA)	Quick Cross	135 cm, 150 cm	2.0F
St Jude	Venture (stopped production recently)	145 cm (rapid exchange), 140 cm (OTW)	2.2F
Terumo	Progreat	110 cm, 130 cm	2.7F
	FineCross MG	130 cm, 150 cm	1.8F
Vascular Solutions	Minnie	90 cm, 135 cm, 150 cm	2.2F
	Gopher	140 cm	3F
	Twin Pass 5200	140 cm	1.9F distal tip, 3F crossing profile
	SuperCross straight and angulated tip (45°, 90°, 120°)	130 cm and 150 cm	1.8F straight, and 2.1F angulated

Data from Brilakis ES, Grantham JA, Thompson CA, et al. The retrograde approach to coronary artery chronic total occlusions. Catheter Cardiovasc Interv 2011;79:3–19.

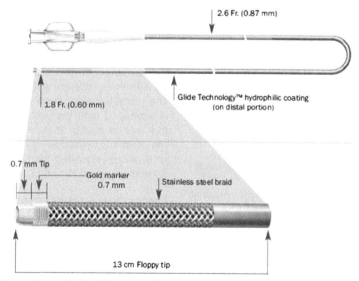

Fig. 5. FineCross microcatheter. Fr, French; mm, millimeter. (*Courtesy of* Terumo Medical Corporation, Somerset, NJ; with permission.)

the crossing profile, while a 1.5 × 15 mm coronary angioplasty balloon provides 7 mm of balloon distal to the marker band that could aid in the gradual push and dilate technique through the occlusion.

Corsair Microcatheters

The Corsair microcatheter is designed for crossing and dilating the collateral channels to facilitate CTO PCI with retrograde techniques.[15] This catheter is formed from tungsten braiding of 10 elliptical stainless steel braids. In addition to superior collateral channel crossing ability, the Corsair microcatheter allows contrast injection and wire exchanges. Because of the Corsair microcatheter lubricity and design it provides good wire manipulation, tactile feedback, and, most important, the ability to track around severely angulated bends.

The Corsair is advanced or retracted OTW with bidirectional rotational movements while the wire is held in the operator's hand to prevent wire rotation and damage.

Tornus Microcatheter

The Tornus microcatheter (Asahi Intecc, Santa Ana, CA, USA) is designed to advance into a lesion with a screw-like technique, when a coronary angioplasty balloon or other microcatheters could not advance OTW. The Tornus microcatheter is made from eight individual stainless steel wires (0.007 in) stranded together to form the microcatheter (**Fig. 6**). Because of its material and design, the Tornus microcatheter provides additional wire support beyond that provided by OTW coronary angioplasty balloons or other commercially available microcatheters (**Fig. 7**).

Tornus 2.1Fr

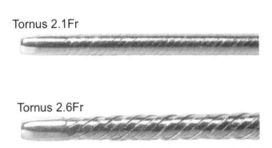

Tornus 2.6Fr

Fig. 6. Tornus microcatheter is made of eight individual wires (0.007 in each) stranded together to form the catheter. Features include OTW system, 135 cm working length, compatible with 0.014 in guide wire only (smallest internal diameter is 0.016 in), 1 mm distal radiopaque marker, and a tapered tip. Because the microcatheter walls are porous it cannot be used for aspiration or infusion. Fr, French. (*Courtesy of* ASAHI Intecc USA, Inc., Santa Ana, CA; with permission.)

The Tornus microcatheter is rotated (screwed in) counterclockwise to advance into the lesion and clockwise for pull back. To protect the integrity of the catheter during use, it is important to relieve the built up tension by counterrotating the catheter 4 clockwise rotations after each 20 counterclockwise turns.

The Tornus catheter used during CTO PCI either opens a larger track for subsequent coronary angioplasty balloon tracking OTW or provides a platform for wire exchange to a more supportive coronary guide wire or to a wire suitable for subsequent rotational atherectomy. Because of its porous design, the Tornus microcatheter cannot be used for infusions or aspirations.

The ability to cross a calcified lesion by the Tornus microcatheters was studied by Fang and colleagues.[16] They found better success rates in crossing the lesion when the calcification was classified as moderate or mild.

Angulated Microcatheter for Angulated Wire Direction

Usually, interventional cardiologists can manipulate the coronary guide wire into a severely angulated side branch or a coronary artery. However, there is a need for angulated support to cross an ostial or proximal CTO in an angulated branch or coronary artery, or when the angulation is more than 90° as in a saphenous vein graft (SVG) anastomosis to a coronary artery.

There are two commercially available microcatheters: the Venture Wire Control catheter (St Jude Medical, St Paul, MN, USA), which provides controlled angulation, and the SuperCross microcatheters (Vascular Solutions, Inc, Minneapolis, MN, USA), which provides passive angulation. The Venture Wire Control catheter has a deflectable distal segment (**Fig. 8**), which is controlled by a proximal tip deflection twist knob. The SuperCross microcatheters are preshaped at the distal tip with three different angles: 45°, 90°, and 120°. The distal tip straightens when the microcatheter is advanced over the coronary guide wire. When the wire is pulled back at the desired location, the catheter restores its preshaped form to provide an angulated platform to direct the wire tip in the desired direction.

DISSECTION AND REENTRY EQUIPMENT

Wire-induced dissection in the subintimal space is the most common mode of CTO PCI failure.[1] Reentry into the true lumen is then attempted using several techniques. Stiff and controlled torque coronary guide wires are usually used to reenter the true lumen, but the subintimal space

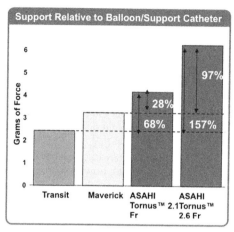

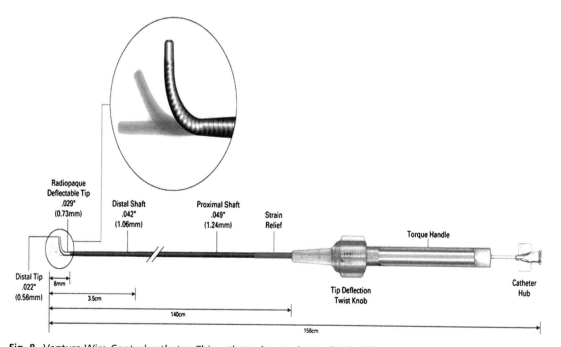

Fig. 7. Comparison of Tornus microcatheter wire support to a Maverick balloon (Boston Scientific, Natick, MA, USA), and Transit 2.5F microcatheter (Cordis, Warren, NJ, USA). (*Courtesy of* ASAHI Intecc USA, Inc., Santa Ana, CA; with permission.)

expands easily and does not provide back-up support to puncture into the true lumen. The subintimal tracking and reentry (STAR) technique is performed by pushing a knuckled polymer-jacketed (see **Fig. 1**) wire until it reenters the true lumen.[17] The STAR technique shears off all the side branches before the reentry point, which could increase the risk of myocardial infarction and cause the loss of collateral channels. A contrast-guided STAR technique uses an injection through a microcatheter pushed inside the proximal occlusion cap to intentionally induce hydrodissection and occasionally hydro-reentry.[18] This technique suffers from the same drawbacks of the STAR technique and is associated with a relatively high risk of complications.

Fig. 8. Venture Wire Control catheter. This catheter has an 8 mm distal deflectable tip, which can be angulated up to 90°. The tip is deflected by twisting the tip deflection twist knob. The Venture Wire Control catheter is available in an OTW and rapid exchange designs. The OTW design is more suitable for CTO PCI. mm, millimeter. (*Courtesy of* St. Jude Medical, Maple Grove, MN; with permission.)

The BridgePoint System

This system is intended to induce a controlled subintimal dissection for subsequent reentry in the true lumen at a desired point (**Figs. 9** and **10**A, C). The introduction of the BridgePoint System (Bridge-Point Medical, Inc., Plymouth, MN, USA) allowed the adoption of dissection and reentry into the true lumen as a primary technique for CTO PCI.

The system has three components: CrossBoss catheter (see **Fig. 9**), Stingray catheter, and Stingray guide wire (see **Fig. 10**A, C).

The CrossBoss CTO Catheter

The CrossBoss catheter (BridgePoint Medical, Inc., Plymouth, MN, USA) provides controlled dissection that can be stopped at a desired reentry point, at or beyond the distal cap of a coronary CTO (see **Fig. 9**). Controlled dissection with the CrossBoss catheter facilitates moving the base of operation from the proximal occlusion CTO cap to a new base of operation if the proximal CTO cap cannot be crossed with wire techniques. Contrary to coronary guide wire loop and hydro dissections, the CrossBoss catheter induces a single subintimal track with a small subintimal space that provides good back up support for the reentry into the true lumen at or beyond the distal CTO cap. The CrossBoss has a multiwire coiled shaft and an OTW design that has a 3.0F nontraumatic rounded tip, with a torquing device. The catheter is advanced over a 0.014 in coronary guide wire to the proximal cap, then the coronary guide wire is pulled back a short distance in the catheter. The catheter is rotated manually as fast as possible, a technique called fast spin. Fast rotations transfer the resistance from the tip of the catheter, which results in the catheter advancing under its own weight. The guide wire is then advanced and the CrossBoss catheter is removed, leaving the guide wire in the subintimal space for the next step of reentry using the Stingray CTO Reentry System (BridgePoint Medical, Inc., Plymouth, MN, USA) or a wire reentry technique.

The CrossBoss catheter crossed intraluminally to the distal true lumen in 30% of the treated lesions during the Facilitated Antegrade Steering Technique in Chronic Total Occlusions (FAST-CTOs) trial.[19] Although in-stent restenosis that resulted in complete occlusions were excluded from the FAST-CTOs trial, the CrossBoss catheter was used successfully to cross the true lumen of totally occluded stents; however, the safety and efficacy of the CrossBoss catheter in CTO inside a coronary stent has not been demonstrated in a clinical trial.

The Stingray CTO Reentry System

The Stingray CTO Reentry System includes a balloon catheter and a guide wire, which are designed to accurately target and reenter the true lumen from the subintimal space (see **Fig. 10**A). The Stingray Balloon Catheter (BridgePoint Medical, Inc., Plymouth, MN, USA) is a self-orienting balloon that becomes flat after inflation at 3 to 4 atmospheres; the balloon has two 180° opposed and offset exit ports in addition to the OTW lumen (see **Fig. 10**B). The Stingray CTO Reentry guide wire has a good control torque and a 28-degree bend at the tip, with a small tip probe that helps in catching and puncturing through the intima to the true lumen (see **Fig. 10**C); the Stingray CTO Reentry guide wire design facilitates exit port selection in the Stingray balloon. Angiographic orthogonal views determine which exit port will direct the wire toward the true vessel lumen. The Stingray wire was used to puncture and gain access to the distal true lumen during the initial experience with the Stingray reentry system. The stiff and sharp tip of the Stingray reentry guide wire frequently induced dissection in the distal vessel. More recently, the wire swap technique is used, whereas the Stingray reentry guide wire is used to puncture a track in the intima, then the wire is replaced with a soft tip polymer-jacketed wire to slip in the true lumen and avoid dissections.

FAST-CTOs Trial

The FAST-CTOs trial was a multicenter non-randomized study to demonstrate the safety and effectiveness of the BridgePoint Medical System in comparison to historical controls.[19] In the United States, 149 patients with a coronary CTO were enrolled in the trial. The patients were included if the coronary CTO was refractory to a conventional guide wire, defined by the following: inability to cross the occlusion after a minimum of 10 min of

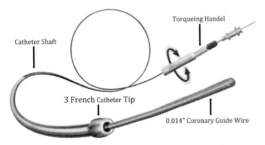

Fig. 9. CrossBoss catheter is part of the BridgePoint System that intended for the performance of controlled subintimal dissection and reentry in the true lumen beyond coronary CTO. (*Courtesy of* BridgePoint Medical, Plymouth, MN; with permission.)

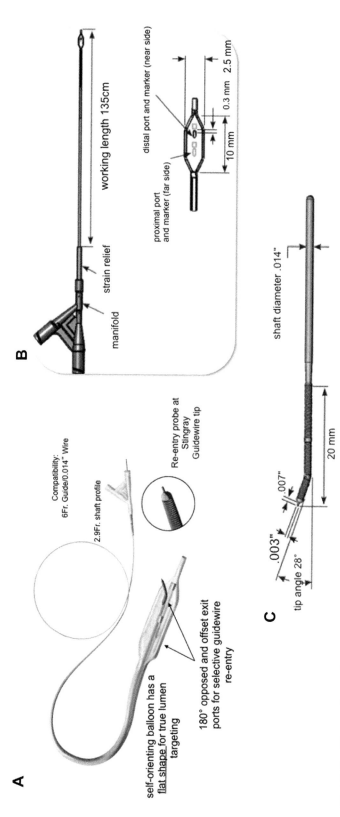

Fig. 10. (*A*) The Stingray System has two components. (*B*) Stingray self-orienting balloon structure. (*C*) Stingray reentry coronary guide wire. Fr, French; mm, millimeter. (*Courtesy of* BridgePoint Medical, Plymouth, MN; with permission.)

fluoroscopy time; a previously failed crossing attempt; or, if best effort attempts result in the conventional guide wire antegrade, advancement into the subintimal plane. Technical success was defined as the ability of the CrossBoss CTO Catheter, Stingray CTO Orienting Balloon Catheter, and/or Stingray Reentry Guide wire to successfully facilitate placement of a guide wire beyond a CTO in the vessel true lumen.

A 77% overall success rate was achieved during the trial. The thirty-day Major adverse coronary events (MACE) rate was 4.8%. These results compared favorably to similarly designed CTO device trials with comparable technical success and safety measures.

The success rate improved with increased experience with the BridgePoint System; the success rate was 70% in the first 74 patients enrolled in the trial, and 86% in patients 75 to 147. The wire swap technique has the potential to increase the success rate beyond the rate achieved in the FAST CTOs trial.

INTRAVASCULAR ULTRASOUND IN CTO PCI

The NATO group members use intravascular ultrasound (IVUS) less frequently than their Japanese colleagues during CTO PCI. The application of IVUS during CTO PCI depends on the local expertise. At this stage of technology development, it is possible to run a successful CTO PCI program without available IVUS.

IVUS over the antegrade coronary guide wire is used to determine if the antegrade or the retrograde wire course is in the true lumen versus a dissection plane. IVUS over a coronary guide wire in a side branch at the proximal cap provides information about the location of the occlusion cap and helps in directing the wire into the true lumen.[20]

Currently, 6F guide catheters cannot accommodate the available IVUS catheters simultaneously with another device. To use IVUS simultaneously with other devices in the same guide catheter, RA operators have to use either a 7F guide catheter if tolerated, or the ping-pong guide catheters technique.

GUIDE CATHETER SUPPORT EQUIPMENT AND TECHNIQUES IN CTO PCI

Additional guide catheter support is frequently needed during CTO PCI, especially when using access from the radial artery. Several techniques are used to enhance guide catheter support (**Box 3**).[21] The first four techniques in **Box 3** are well described in the literature and are applied

---

> **Box 3**
> **Techniques to enhance guide catheter support during CTO PCI**
>
> Guide catheter deep intubation in the coronary artery tree
>
> Large guide catheters (frequently not possible from the radial artery)
>
> Buddy and anchoring wire techniques
>
> Anchoring angioplasty balloon technique
>
> Mother and child guide catheters technique

---

using the usually available devices in every catheterization laboratory that routinely performs PCI.

The mother-and-child guide catheter technique depends on the support provided by the introduction of another catheter (child) through the guide catheter (mother). The child catheter is extended in the proximal segment of the coronary artery over the coronary guide wire (**Fig. 11**). The introduction of a less traumatic child catheter provides more support and coaxial engagement regardless of the mother guide catheter shape (**Fig. 12**). The use of a child catheter during CTO PCI provides several other useful functions (**Box 4**), including lowering the contrast load and stent protection during delivery to the lesion.[22]

There are three commercially available catheters that can be used as a child catheter inside the mother guide catheter; the Proxis device (St Jude Medical, St Paul, MN, USA) that is designed for proximal occlusion of an SVG to provide distal embolic protection during catheter interventions on an SVG, the Heartrail catheters (Heartrail, Terumo, Japan) (**Fig. 13**),[23] and the GuideLiner catheters (Vascular Solution, Minneapolis, MN, USA) (**Fig. 14**), which has a rapid exchange design whereas the first two have an OTW design. The GuideLiner can be used with standard PCI equipment, but it results in an internal diameter approximately 1F smaller than the mother guide catheter. The GuideLiner catheters are available in three sizes: 6Fr, 7Fr, and 8Fr.

The GuideLiner is passed through the hemostatic valve over a guide wire. The GuideLiner catheters should not be advanced in vessels less than 2.5 mm and the distal end should not extend more than 10 cm out of the mother guide catheter.

WIRE EXTERNALIZATION TECHNIQUES AND EQUIPMENT

Wire externalization of the retrograde guide wire allows access to both ends of the coronary guide wire and provides excellent support for coronary

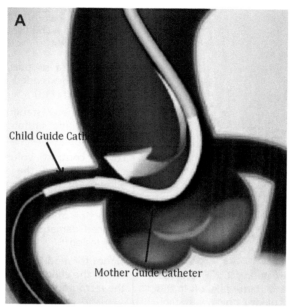

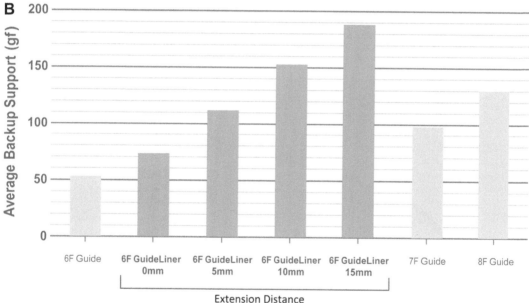

Fig. 11. (*A*) Mother-and-child guide catheters technique. The child catheter extends in the proximal segment of the coronary artery to enhance the support of the mother guide catheter and provide coaxial engagement in the coronary artery ostium. (*B*) GuideLiner support according to distance extended in the coronary artery; with 15 mm of extension, the 6F in a 6F guide catheter provides backup support superior to an 8F guide catheter. F, French; gf, gram force; mm, millimeter. (*Courtesy of* Vascular Solution Inc., Minneapolis, MN; with permission.)

gear delivery. The retrograde wire can incidentally or intentionally enter the antegrade guide catheter after retrogradely crossing the collateral circulation and the CTO lesion. A longer guide wire is frequently needed if the wire used to retrogradely cross the CTO lesion is 300 cm or shorter, especially when the guide catheters are longer than 90 cm. The retrograde wire can be pinned in the antegrade guide catheter by an inflated coronary angioplasty balloon. The rail provided by the pinned retrograde coronary wire facilitates the advancement of the retrograde microcatheter to the antegrade guide catheter. Placement of the retrograde microcatheter tip in the antegrade guide catheter provides a platform for wire exchange to a longer wire for externalization from the antegrade hemostatic valve (see **Box 2**).

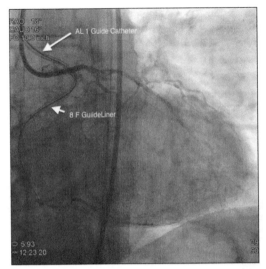

Fig. 12. Coronary angiogram during RCA CTO revascularization. The RCA has an anterior take off in this patient, the 8F AL1 (mother) guide catheter was stabilized in the RCA ostium with an 8F GuideLiner (child) catheter introduced over a coronary guide wire to the mid-RCA segment. (*Courtesy of* Vascular Solution Inc., Minneapolis, MN; with permission.)

Box 4
Functions of a child catheter in a mother guide catheter in PCI

Provide extra support, which correlates with the length extended in the coronary artery tree (see **Fig. 11B**)

Guide catheter stabilization, especially if the mother guide catheter cannot provide good coaxial engagement (see **Fig. 12**).

Lower contrast volume, deep or selective engagement in the branch coronary vessel allows for lower contrast volume during angiography

Protection of drug-eluting stents from friction-induced damage during delivery to the coronary lesion[22]

Target for modified reverse CART technique; in which the child catheter is used as a target for the retrograde coronary guide wire.

Abbreviation: CART, controlled antegrade and retrograde subintimal tracking.

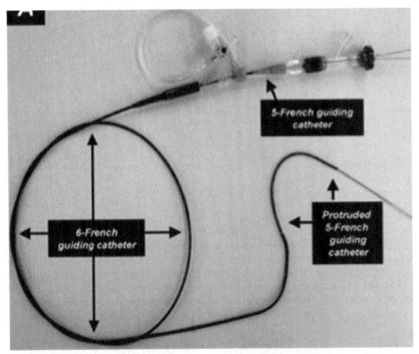

Fig. 13. Mother-and child-guide catheter model using the Heartrail (Heartrail, Terumo, Japan). The 5F Heartrail straight-guiding catheter is 120 cm, whereas the 6F guiding catheter is 100 cm. The 5F Heartrail catheter has a very soft 13 cm end portion, which can easily negotiate the tortuous coronary artery with minimal damage and then be inserted more deeply into the artery. The inner lumen of the 5F Heartrail catheter has an 0.059 in diameter; it can accept normal balloons or stent delivery systems less than 4.0 mm in diameter. The inner lumen of the outer 6F guide catheter must be more than 0.071′ in diameter to accommodate the 5F Heartrail catheter. (*From* Takahashi S, Saito S, Tanaka S, et al. New method to increase a backup support of a 6 French guiding coronary catheter. Catheter Cardiovasc Interv 2004;63:452–6; with permission.)

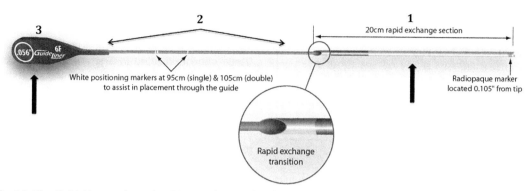

Fig. 14. The GuideLiner catheter is a 20 cm soft-tipped catheter (1) connected via a metal collar (magnified inlet) to a 115 cm stainless steel shaft (2) with a large proximal tab (3) for accurate positioning of the device within the coronary system. cm, centimeter. (*Courtesy of* Vascular Solution Inc., Minneapolis, MN; with permission.)

When the retrograde wire cannot be directed to enter the antegrade guide catheter, a snare device is used to capture and exteriorize the wire from the hemostatic valve. Snares are wire-based devices that use the noose technique to capture and remove wires or catheters in the circulation (**Fig. 15**). Snares come in different models and sizes that allow wire capturing in the coronary artery tree or in the aorta. Because the space is more limited it is easier to snare the wire end in the aortic arch than the aortic root.

The most commonly used snares in the United States are the EN snares (Merit Medical Systems, Inc, South Jordan, UT, USA) and Goose Neck snares (ev3 Endovascular, Inc, Plymouth, MN, USA). The EN Snare is an interlaced Nitinol loop that looks like a tulip that maximizes the chance of capturing the wire end (see **Fig. 15**). The size chosen when capturing the retrograde wire in the aorta is 12 to 20 mm with 6F guide catheters, and 18 to 30 mm with 7F or 8F guide catheters. The snare sizes for capturing the wire in the coronary arteries are 2 to 4 mm or 4 to 6 mm. Amplatz

GooseNeck snares (ev3 Endovascular, Inc., Plymouth, MN, USA) are formed with one loop that forms a true 90° angle with the snare shaft, thus making the device remain coaxial to the lumen.

COMPLICATIONS MANAGEMENT EQUIPMENT

Complication prevention strategies are an important part of the skill set necessary for a successful CTO PCI procedure. However, complications management equipment should be available in every catheterization laboratory performing PCI (**Box 5**). Because CTO PCI operators use new techniques, new and unfamiliar situations are arising during CTO PCI. Initial temporary control of the complication, and regrouping and thinking through the potential solutions, are the most important steps in the management of any complication. Coronary perforations are managed according to their severity location and inducing device.

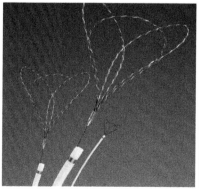

EN Snare

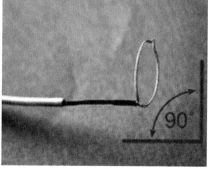

GooseNeck Snare

Fig. 15. En Snare (Merit Medical Systems, Inc., South Jordan, UT, USA). GooseNeck (ev3 Endovascular, Inc. Plymouth, MN, USA). (EN Snare® Endovascular Snare System image *courtesy of* Merit Medical, South Jordan, UT; with permission. Gooseneck Snare image *courtesy of* ev3 Endovascular, Plymouth, MN; with permission.)

Coils and injectable material are used for an end branch wire perforation. A special delivery catheter might be required for delivery of the coils or the injectable martial. The 0.014 in coils are not widely available in catheterization laboratories that do not perform neurointerventions. Most 0.014 in coils are detachable, more expensive than pushable coils, and require more training, whereas 0.018 in coils are widely available and easier to deliver by simple push technique. Radiologists use injectable material (particles and glue) to induce arteriovenous malformations thrombosis.

The injectable particles should be larger or should clump together to become larger than the perforation defect. The patient's own clotted blood or fat tissue can be injected in a small branch to seal a wire-induced perforation. When injecting material in a perforated coronary artery branch, care must be taken to prevent spilling the injectable material in other coronary arteries or branches by inflating a coronary angioplasty balloon proximal to the injection site, or injecting through the distal lumen of an inflated OTW coronary angioplasty balloon.

JoStent grafts (Abbott Laboratories, Abbott Park, IL, USA) are used to seal a vessel rupture, which is usually induced by an angioplasty balloon or a stent deployment. The JoStent graft is made of two stents with an expandable polytetrafluoroethylene graft material wrapped between them. The JoStent grafts in the United States are OTW and require at least 7F guide catheters, whereas rapid exchange JoStent grafts are available outside the United States and can be delivered through a 6F guide catheter.

Table 5
The parsimonious CTO PCI toolbox[a]

Tool	Quantity and Specifications
Sheaths	Six large-bore 7–8F, 45–55 cm long
Guide catheters	Five 8F and 6F 90 cm long in each of the following configurations with and without side holes: Judkins Right 4, Amplatz Left 1 and 0.75, and Launcher EBU 3.75, 4, and 4.5
Coronary guide wires	Five of each of the following wires: Fielder FC, Fielder XT, Pilot 200, Confianza Pro-12, Pilot 50, Viper wire advance
Microcatheters	Five OTW coronary angioplasty balloons (1.5 mm or smaller) Two FineCross 150 cm microcatheters
Child catheters for mother-and-child guide catheter technique	Four of each of the 6F and 8F GuideLiner catheters
Tornus	Two 2.6F Two 2.1F
Corsair microcatheters	Five of the 150 cm long Corsair microcatheters
Angulated access microcatheters	Two Venture wire control or Two 120° SuperCross
En snares	Two of 12–20 mm and 18–30 mm
BridgePoint System for controlled dissection and reentry (CrossBoss, Stingray Balloon, Stingray wire)	Five complete systems
Coils and delivery system	Two of either 0.018 in or 0.014 in
JoStent graft	One of commercially available size

[a] The minimum amount of equipment kept in the Appleton Medical Center (Appleton, WI, USA) catheterization laboratory since the beginning of the CTO PCI program—not including equipment available in most catheterization laboratories that routinely perform PCI.

SUMMARY

CTO PCI is gaining more popularity and familiarity among interventional cardiologists. Learning the skills necessary to improve CTO PCI success rate to above 90% requires a systematic plan to learn the techniques and gain the experience in CTO PCI. A few devices must be available in the catheterization laboratory to insure successful and safe CTO PCI procedures. The CTO PCI toolbox is not significantly more expensive than the non–CTO PCI toolbox. A list of the inventory required in the CTO PCI toolbox is provided in **Table 5**.

REFERENCES

1. Stone GW, Reifart NJ, Moussa I, et al. Percutaneous recanalization of chronically occluded coronary arteries: a consensus document: part II. Circulation 2005;112:2530–7.
2. Grantham JA, Marso SP, Spertus J, et al. Chronic total occlusion angioplasty in the United States. JACC Cardiovasc Interv 2009;2:479–86.
3. Christofferson RD, Lehmann KG, Martin GV, et al. Effect of chronic total coronary occlusion on treatment strategy. Am J Cardiol 2005;95:1088–91.
4. Serruys PW. SYNTAX trial: chronic total occlusion subsets. Oral presentation at: Cardiovascular Research Technologies 2009. Washington DC; 2009.
5. Serruys PW, Morice MC, Kappetein AP, et al. Percutaneous coronary intervention versus coronary-artery bypass grafting for severe coronary artery disease. N Engl J Med 2009;360:961–72.
6. Thompson CA. Percutaneous revascularization of coronary chronic total occlusions: the new era begins. JACC Cardiovasc Interv 2010;3:152–4.
7. Sumitsuji S, Inoue K, Ochiai M, et al. Fundamental wire technique and current standard strategy of percutaneous intervention for chronic total occlusion with histopathological insights. JACC Cardiovasc Interv 2011;4:941–51.
8. Morino Y, Kimura T, Hayashi Y, et al. In-hospital outcomes of contemporary percutaneous coronary intervention in patients with chronic total occlusion: insights from the J-CTO registry (Multicenter CTO Registry in Japan). JACC Cardiovasc Interv 2010; 3:143–51.
9. Thompson CA, Jayne JE, Robb JF, et al. Retrograde techniques and the impact of operator volume on percutaneous intervention for coronary chronic total occlusions: an early U.S. experience. JACC Cardiovasc Interv 2009;2:834–42.
10. Brilakis ES, Grantham JA, Thompson CA, et al. The retrograde approach to coronary artery chronic total occlusions. Catheter Cardiovasc Interv 2011;79:3–19.
11. Cantor WJ, Mahaffey KW, Huang Z, et al. Bleeding complications in patients with acute coronary syndrome undergoing early invasive management can be reduced with radial access, smaller sheath sizes, and timely sheath removal. Catheter Cardiovasc Interv 2007;69:73–83.
12. Brueck M, Bandorski D, Kramer W, et al. A randomized comparison of transradial versus transfemoral approach for coronary angiography and angioplasty. JACC Cardiovasc Interv 2009;2:1047–54.
13. Brilakis ES, Grantham JA, Banerjee S. "Ping-pong" guide catheter technique for retrograde intervention of a chronic total occlusion through an ipsilateral collateral. Catheter Cardiovasc Interv 2011;78:395–9.
14. Ron Waksman SS. Chronic total occlusion book: a guide to recanalization. West Sussex (UK): Blackwell; 2009.
15. Tsuchikane E, Katoh O, Kimura M, et al. The first clinical experience with a novel catheter for collateral channel tracking in retrograde approach for chronic coronary total occlusions. JACC Cardiovasc Interv 2010;3:165–71.
16. Fang HY, Lee CH, Fang CY, et al. Application of penetration device (Tornus) for percutaneous coronary intervention in balloon uncrossable chronic total occlusion—procedure outcomes, complications, and predictors of device success. Catheter Cardiovasc Interv 2011;78:356–62.
17. Colombo A, Mikhail GW, Michev I, et al. Treating chronic total occlusions using subintimal tracking and reentry: the STAR technique. Catheter Cardiovasc Interv 2005;64:407–11.
18. Carlino M, Latib A, Godino C, et al. CTO recanalization by intraocclusion injection of contrast: the microchannel technique. Catheter Cardiovasc Interv 2008;71:20–6.
19. Wyman RM. The BridgePoint Medical CTO System: results of the "FAST-CTO" US IDE Study. Oral presentation at: Trans Catheter Therapeutics. Washington DC; 2010.
20. Matsubara T, Murata A, Kanyama H, et al. IVUS-guided wiring technique: promising approach for the chronic total occlusion. Catheter Cardiovasc Interv 2004;61:381–6.
21. Di Mario C, Ramasami N. Techniques to enhance guide catheter support. Catheter Cardiovasc Interv 2008;72:505–12.
22. Kuriyama N, Kobayashi Y, Yamaguchi M, et al. Usefulness of rotational atherectomy in preventing polymer damage of everolimus-eluting stent in calcified coronary artery. JACC Cardiovasc Interv 2011; 4:588–9.
23. Takahashi S, Saito S, Tanaka S, et al. New method to increase a backup support of a 6 French guiding coronary catheter. Catheter Cardiovasc Interv 2004;63:452–6.

CTO PCI Procedural Planning

Nicholas J. Lembo, MD*, Dimitri Karmpaliotis, MD,
David E. Kandzari, MD

KEYWORDS

- Chronic total occlusion • Coronary artery disease • Percutaneous coronary intervention
- Iodinated contrast • Radiation exposure

KEY POINTS

- Revascularization decisions in patients with coronary chronic total occlusions (CTO) are complex and multifactorial, representing a balance of clinical and procedural risk and benefit.
- Careful preprocedural angiographic assessment is a key to successful CTO percutaneous coronary intervention (PCI).
- CTO PCI may require greater utilization of iodinated contrast, presenting a higher risk of contrast-induced kidney disease; consideration of risk of nephropathy and measures to prevent its occurrence are essential.
- Patient and operator radiation exposure is significantly increased during CTO PCI and steps need to be taken to minimize exposure.
- Given the complexity of CTO PCI, specific training is required for both operators and catheterization laboratory staff.

INTRODUCTION

Chronic total occlusion percutaneous coronary intervention (CTO PCI) procedural planning involves much thought and deliberation before one actually attempts to cross the CTO lesion in the cardiac catheterization laboratory. One must first decide whether or not to revascularize a CTO vessel based on patient and myocardial viability issues. A key factor is the preprocedural angiographic assessment of the CTO vessel and collateral filling. Procedural pharmacology guidelines also must be followed closely. In addition, secondary to the potential risks of complications, CTO PCI generally requires significantly more contrast and radiation. Both preprocedure and postprocedure management are essential. Dual access and guide catheter length and support are also important for procedural success. Finally, CTO PCI represents the most complex PCI one can perform and thus operator and staff training as well as the concept of CTO days are all essential for a successful CTO PCI program.

REVASCULARIZATION STRATEGIES

The decision to revascularize a patient with coronary CTO is complex and multifactorial. It includes patient characteristics and comorbidities, such as age, symptoms, renal function, ability to take long-term dual antiplatelet therapy, previous cardiac radiation exposure, weight, ability to have dual vascular access sties, and a willingness of the operator to appropriately prepare for the procedure when compared with standard non-CTO PCI. Angiographic features of the CTO, although important to the "beginner" CTO operator, become less important to the high-volume CTO operator. This is discussed in detail in other articles in this issue.

One needs to carefully weigh the risk/benefit ratio from all PCI revascularization procedures; CTO PCI is no different. With considerate assessment of CTO procedural strategy, patients will receive substantial clinical benefit through relief of symptoms refractory to medical therapy, reduction of ischemia burden identified by noninvasive imaging and/or improvement in left ventricular function.

Piedmont Heart Institute, 275 Collier Road North West, Suite 300, Atlanta, GA 30309, USA
* Corresponding author.
E-mail address: Nicholas.Lembo@piedmont.org

Intervent Cardiol Clin 1 (2012) 299–308
doi:10.1016/j.iccl.2012.04.002
2211-7458/12/$ – see front matter © 2012 Published by Elsevier Inc.

ASSESSING FOR VIABLE MYOCARDIUM

The assessment of viable hibernating myocardium versus transmurally infarcted myocardium is important in determining whether CTO PCI revascularization will be beneficial to the patient. Exposing a patient to risks of CTO PCI with irreversibly damaged myocardium is never warranted. Similarly, not offering CTO PCI in patients with viable hibernating myocardium is withholding therapy in patients who may be most in need.

A simple assessment can be presence or absence of Q-waves on the 12-lead electrocardiogram in the distribution of the CTO, to assess myocardial viability. The absence of Q-waves in the distribution of CTO generally is associated with hibernating myocardium that should improve with revascularization. Conversely, presence of the Q-waves may more often be associated with transmurally infarcted myocardium in which CTO revascularization may not improve left ventricular function.[1]

Myocardial perfusion imaging may be used to assess myocardial viability in patients with severe wall motion abnormalities in the distribution of the CTO. Patients with delayed uptake on rest-redistribution at 24 hours is associated with myocardial cellular activity and again would benefit from revascularization. Conversely, no delayed reuptake is associated with irreversibly injured myocardium, and patients would therefore not derive benefit from CTO revascularization.[2]

The present nuclear cardiology gold standard to assess myocardial viability is positron emission tomography (PET). Patients with CTOs in the distribution of severe wall motion abnormalities who have low blood flow perfusion and high metabolic update will generally demonstrate improved left ventricular function after successful CTO PCI revascularization. Patients with low blood flow perfusion in the absence of metabolic uptake will not improve left ventricular function despite successful CTO PCI revascularization.[3]

Magnetic resonance imaging (MRI) is an excellent tool to assess myocardial perfusion, myocardial viability, contractile reserve, and cardiac metabolism in a patient's severe wall motion abnormalities in the distribution of the CTO vessel. Cardiac MRI is thought to be superior to single-photon emission tomography and PET imaging for detecting hibernating myocardium that will show improvement in wall motion after CTO revascularization.[4]

PREPROCEDURAL ANGIOGRAPHIC ASSESSMENT

The preprocedure assessment of the coronary angiogram is essential to successful strategy planning in CTO revascularization, and requires significant time in reviewing the angiogram. Thus, we do not recommend ad hoc PCI for CTO lesions. Unfortunately, many of these coronary angiograms are performed by noninterventional or non-CTO interventional cardiologists who look at angiograms in a much different manner than does a CTO interventionist. We therefore need to train our angiographic colleagues on proper CTO angiographic techniques, as described in this article.

CTO Vessel

Angiography of the CTO vessel is a key component in deciding on the technique for CTO revascularization. It is key to determining all the features of the CTO, which can best be determined by ipsilateral and contralateral simultaneous injections. For successful antegrade CTO revascularization, one needs to penetrate the proximal cap, traverse the length of the CTO body, and exit the distal cap into the true lumen.[5]

Angiographic assessment of proximal cap features include tapered versus blunt appearance, sidebranch involvement, calcification, bridging collaterals and presence or absence of a microchannel. Tapered or beaked appearance of the proximal cap is a favorable angiographic finding compared with convex or blunt proximal caps. Absence of side branches is also favorable, as is the lack of calcifications. The key feature is to know where the ongoing vessel is, ie, no anatomic ambiguity; if so, an antegrade approach is favored. If the proximal cap has anatomic ambiguity, then a retrograde approach will be favored.

Angiographic assessment of the CTO body should be carefully assessed. This should include estimation of the length, tortuosity, calcification, presence of bridging collaterals, microchannels, and anatomic path of the vessel. Patients with anatomic ambiguity of a long CTO occlusion may be better approached with a dissection and reentry strategy rather than guidewire attempts to maintain a luminal course through the entire segment.

The distal cap should also be carefully assessed with regard to the presence of the distal vessel target size and whether the distal cap is at a bifurcation. To fully assess the proximal cap, CTO body, and distal cap, simultaneous bilateral angiography should be performed in multiple projections.

Other features to be assessed on the procedure angiogram include proximal vessel tortuosity, side branches arising from the CTO body, distal vessel disease, previous bypass graft insertion sites, ostial location sites, and disease in the donor collateral vessel, which could be problematic when passing gear retrograde.

Contralateral Injections

Except for CTO vessels, which are supplied only by ipsilateral collaterals, the use of bilateral injections is essential in the successful performance of CTO PCI revascularization. The key to successful contralateral angiography is to identify collaterals with no panning and a magnification in which all collaterals and vessels are visualized and prolonged imaging exposure. On occasion, contralateral collaterals may have 2 sources, ie, native vessel and a bypass graft. Thus, on rare occasions one may need more than 2 arterial access sites to properly visualize retrograde filling of a CTO.

It is strongly recommended that bilateral arterial access sites are obtained before the administration of parenteral anticoagulation, thereby avoiding an arterial stick in a fully anticoagulated patient. It is also recommended that if a CTO interventionist is performing the diagnostic catheterization, the maximal amount of angiographic information be obtained at that time and includes bilateral injections.

In general, one should inject the vessel in which the collaterals arise and after a 2-second delay inject the CTO vessel. Bridging collaterals are important to recognize and avoid during both antegrade and retrograde crossing attempts to minimize the risk of perforation, especially when advancing microcatheters and balloons. Septal collaterals arising from the right coronary artery (RCA) to the left anterior descending (LAD) or from the LAD to the RCA are usually best visualized in the right anterior oblique (RAO) cranial view. Epicardial collaterals vary in course and customized views are often needed. Collaterals between obtuse marginal and posterolateral branches and diagonal to obtuse marginal branches can best be seen in left anterior oblique (LAO) and RAO cranial projections. Collaterals between the proximal obtuse marginal and the right coronary artery are often seen in RAO and anteroposterior caudal projections.

CARDIOVASCULAR COMPUTED TOMOGRAPHY ANGIOGRAPHY

Multislice contrasted enhanced cardiovascular computed tomography angiography (CTA) may be helpful in certain patients with complex CTO anatomy or previously failed attempts by an experienced CTO interventionist. Cardiac CTA may therefore be helpful with ostial occlusions, ambiguous vessel courses, anomalous take-off vessels, or insertions of occluded bypass grafts to understand previous failure.[6,7]

New computer software systems can now bring the CTA into the catheterization laboratory and co-register the CTA image with the fluoroscopy cine images using the same angulation, thereby allowing the CTO operator to see CTA and live images simultaneously.

Secondary to added contrast load, radiation exposure, and cost, we do not recommend cardiac CTA before all CTO procedures, but it may be useful for complex anatomy or previous failures.

PREPROCEDURAL PHARMACOLOGY

Patients being scheduled for CTO revascularization will almost always be elective; however, exceptions may include patients with acute myocardial infarction with acutely occluded bypass in which CTO PCI of the native vessel is indicated or patients who remain in cardiogenic shock after opening the infarct-related artery. Thus, patients undergoing elective procedures should be on dual antiplatelet therapy customary to the local practice patterns with oral aspirin therapy and adenosine diphosphate inhibitors before scheduling the CTO procedure. The use of glycoprotein IIb/IIIa platelet inhibitors and nonreversible anticoagulants, such as bivalirudin, is not advisable secondary to the potential risk of uncontrolled bleeding in rare instances of coronary perforation and development of tamponade.

PROCEDURAL ANTICOAGULATION

Unfractionated heparin administered intravenously or intra-arterially is the anticoagulant of choice for CTO PCI, secondary to its reversibility with protamine sulfate. Initially a bolus of 80 U/kg of heparin is initiated with the goal activated clotting time (ACT) for antegrade cases of 250 seconds; however, if retrograde PCI is being performed, the goal ACT is 350 seconds to lower the risk of donor vessel thrombosis. If the ACT is not in the therapeutic range, additional heparin is administrated and a repeat ACT should be checked in 5 minutes. Once the ACT is in the therapeutic range, ie, 250 seconds for antegrade cases and 350 seconds for retrograde cases, ACTs should be checked every 30 minutes with a timer in the catheterization laboratory.

CONTRAST LOAD

In general, patients undergoing CTO PCI will require significantly more contrast than those undergoing non-CTO PCI. Thus, the risk of the contrast-induced nephropathy (CIN) is likely higher in patients undergoing CTO PCI. Most studies define CIN as either a relative increase in the serum creatinine of 25% or more above the baseline valve, or an absolute increase of more than 0.5 mg/dL. CIN generally occurs 24 to 48 hours after contrast exposure, peaking at 3 to 5 days and generally returning to baseline after 7 to 10 days. Therefore, careful attention needs to be placed on assessing patients at risk for CIN and preprocedure, procedure, and postprocedure management.

Risk Factors for CIN

The primary risk factory for development of CIN is preexisting renal insufficiency, which is magnified in the presence of diabetes mellitus. Other nonmodifiable risks include congestive heart failure (left ventricular ejection fraction <40%), advanced age (>75 years), and prior transplant, such as renal or cardiac. Modifiable risk factors for CIN include preprocedure dehydration often related to diuretic usage. Nephrotoxic drugs, such as nonsteroidal anti-inflammatory drugs (NSAIDs), cyclosporine, vancomycin, and amphotericin, should be stopped 24 hours before the CTO procedure. Although not nephrotoxic, metformin should be held 48 hours before the 48 hours after contrast to avoid the risk of lactic acidosis if CIN were to occur. Anemia is also an independent predictor of CIN. In addition, recent contrast procedures significantly increase the risk of CIN.[8]

Assessment of Glomerular Filtration Rate

It is recommended that the glomerular filtration rate (GFR) is a more accurate measure of kidney function as compared with serum creatinine. Calculating from serum creatinine alone may be misleading secondary to differences in muscle mass among patients; women and the elderly may have a normal creatinine despite having a low GFR. The American Heart Association has given a Class I indication for the estimation of GFR using the Modification of Diet in Renal Disease (MDRD) equation. Values lower than 60 mL/dL/1.73 m² should be considered abnormal; these patients are at high risk for nephropathy and serum creatinine should be measured 24 to 48 hours after contrast administration. MDRD study equations for calculating GFR are shown in **Fig. 1**.[9]

Choice of Contrast Agent

High-osmolar contrast media, such as diatrizoate and metrizoate, which are generally no longer used, were associated with a significant risk of allergic reactions and nephrotoxicity in patients. Low-osmolar contrast media as compared with high-osmolar contrast media has been shown to be significantly less nephrotoxic, especially in patients with chronic kidney disease, particularly in those with diabetes.[10]

Iso-osmolar contrast media, such as iodixanol, as compared with low-osmolar contrast media, has been shown in a pooled analysis of 16 double-blind comparative trials to have the lowest risk of CIN, especially in those with baseline chronic kidney disease and those with chronic kidney disease and diabetes.[11]

STRATEGIES TO PREVENT CIN

It may seem obvious, but one of the most important strategies to prevent CIN is to have a good understanding of who is at risk and to modify correctable factors.

Pre-PCI Discontinuation of Potentially Toxic Drugs

Potentially nephrotoxic drugs, such as NSAIDs, cyclosporine, vancomycin, and amphotericin, should be withheld 24 hours before contrast administration. Also, metformin should be held for 48 hours before and 48 hours after contrast administration.

MDRD 1 GFR = 170 x [SCr]$^{-0.999}$ x [Age]$^{-0.176}$ x [0.762 if patient is female] x [1.18 if patient is black] x [BUN]$^{-0.170}$ x [Alb]$^{0.318}$

MDRD 2 (Abbreviated) GFR = 186 x [SCr]$^{-1.154}$ x [Age]$^{-0.203}$ x [0.742 if patient is female] x [1.21 if patient is black]

Fig. 1. MDRD study equations for calculating glomerular filtration rate. Alb, serum albumin; BUN, blood urea nitrogen; SCr, serum creatinine. (*From* Brosius FC 3rd, Hostetter TH, Kelepouris E, et al. Detection of chronic kidney disease in patients with or at increased risk of cardiovascular disease; a science advisory from the American Heart Association Kidney And Cardiovascular Disease Council; the Councils on High Blood Pressure Research, Cardiovascular Disease in the Young, and Epidemiology and Prevention; and the Quality of Care and Outcomes Research Interdisciplinary Working Group: developed in collaboration with the National Kidney Foundation. Circulation 2006;114:1083–7; with permission.)

Volume Expansion

Intravascular volume expansion before contrast administration is beneficial secondary to its increasing renal blood flow, decreasing vasoconstriction, and improving tubular filtration. In patients with a low GFR, administration of 1.0 to 1.5 mL/kg per hour of intravenous (IV) isotonic crystalloid should be initiated 12 hours before the procedure and continued for 6 to 24 hours. Outpatients should receive hydration up to 3 hours before and up to 12 hours following the procedure. These recommendations may need to be modified in patients with left ventricular dysfunction and/or congestive heart failure. Sodium bicarbonate protocols have been also been used for prevention of CIN.

N-acetylcysteine is no longer recommended as an agent to prevent CIN and is a Class III indication in the recently described PCI guidelines.[12]

In patients with severe kidney disease, with an estimated GFR of 30 mL per minute or less, one needs to strongly consider the risk/benefit ratio of CTO PCI. Furthermore, nephrology consultation preprocedure is strongly recommended.

These authors also recommend assessment of left ventricular end-diastolic pressure (LVEDP) at the time of CTO PCI to accurately assess the patient's volume status. If the LVEDP is low, one can administer IV fluids to obtain adequate volume expansion before the administration of contrast.

Maximum Recommended Contrast Dose

Because CTO PCI generally uses more contrast than non-CTO PCI, it is essential to try to minimize contrast administration during the CTO procedure. One simple way is to obtain as much information as possible at the time of the diagnostic angiogram. This includes angiographic features of the proximal cap, CTO body, and distal cap, and estimation of length, tortuosity, calcification, bridging collaterals, microchannels, side branches, and course of collateral circulation. This information is best obtained by dual injections at the time of the diagnostic catheterization. Furthermore, the CTO PCI strategy can be formulated, as well as the best angiographic views for the CTO procedure. We also must teach invasive noninterventional and non-CTO interventional colleagues what we are looking for, so they can provide the maximal information from the diagnostic cardiac catheterization. Therefore, having the maximal information will lessen the contrast load at the time of the elective CTO procedure.

A formula based on registry data has been developed for calculating the maximum recommended contrast dose (MRCD).

$$MRCD = [5 \text{ mL of contrast} \times \text{body weight (kg)}] / \text{serum creatinine (mg/dL)}$$

An alternative calculation of the MRCD utilizes creatinine clearance

$$\text{Creatinine Clearance, mL/min} = \frac{(140 - \text{age}) \times \text{Body Weight [kg]}^*}{\text{Serum Creatinine (mg/dL)} \times 72}$$

*Multiply by 0.8 in females

$$MRCD = 6 \times \text{creatinine clearance (mL)}$$

The incidence of CIN requiring dialysis was 2.4% in patients exceeding the MRCD and 0.2% in patients below the MRCD.[13]

Our laboratory calculates MRCD on all of our patients undergoing PCI. The total volume of contrast administered to the patient and the MRCD is reported to the CTO operator every 30 minutes of the procedure along with the total Gy and ACT. The cumulative contrast volume and total Gy also help the operator in strategizing the procedure, changing plans, and changing angiographic views, as well as when the procedure should be terminated.

Postprocedure Management

Postprocedure volume administration is also important in patients with low GFR and is often overlooked. Administration of 1.0 to 1.5 mL/kg per hour of IV isotonic crystalloid should be continued for 6 to 24 hours after PCI. Patients should also be encouraged to drink fluids after the procedure. These recommendations may need to be modified in patients with left ventricular dysfunction or congestive heart failure. It is also important to monitor creatinine levels after the procedure for 24 to 72 hours. If there is evidence of CIN, as defined by an increase in serum creatinine of 25% or more above baseline or an absolute increase more than 0.5 mg/dL the day after the procedure, we continue IV fluid hydration, consider nephrology consultation, and continue monitoring of creatinine.

RADIATION EXPOSURE

Patient and operator radiation exposure is significantly increased in patients undergoing CTO PCI as compared with non-CTO PCI. In our laboratory, patient radiation exposure is the primary reason for termination of the CTO procedure. Thus, careful attention should be made to minimize radiation exposure to the patient as well as to the operator and the staff.[14]

It is also important to assess prior radiation exposure to the patient. For example, if a 3-hour CTO PCI done in one view was attempted 2 weeks earlier, the reattempt should be deferred for a couple of months, paying close attention to whether a radiation burn has occurred.

Biologic Injury

There are 2 main biologic risks of ionizing radiation: deterministic and stochastic.

Deterministic "dose" risk is the amount of radiation absorbed by a particular mass of tissue, such as the skin at the point of beam entry, and measured in units of Gray (Gy) or milliGray (mGy). Skin erythema and ulceration are deterministic effects.

Stochastic "effective" risk measures the effect on the radiated cells that are not killed but have their DNA modified. Effective doses are expressed in Sieverts (Sv) or milliSieverts (mSv).

Deterministic Injury

Skin injury is the most common deterministic effect of radiation to patients in the cardiac catheterization laboratory. Skin cells divide continuously and thus are susceptible to injury at the beam entrance port. The threshold for detecting skin injury with mild redness is about 2 Gy. Skin doses higher than 15 Gy will cause serious injury.

Radiation skin injury may begin a few hours after exposure, with redness and itching that resolves in 1 to 2 days. The full extent of the injury may not become visible for weeks or months after exposure and includes dermal atrophy, telangiectasia, fibrosis, keratosis, hyperpigmentation, depigmentation, chronic ulceration, and pain.

The Joint Commission on Accreditation of Healthcare Organizations has added fluoroscopic skin dose of 15 Gy to the list of sentinel events, which is equivalent to amputating the wrong limb.

Minimizing Radiation Exposure

ALARA (as low as reasonably achievable) should be used as the guiding principle for anyone using x-rays. The interventional cardiologist controls the amount of radiation delivered with the exception of patient size. Patient size is a key factor in radiation exposure, with obesity being a major risk factor for skin injury. For each centimeter of tissue, the input dose is increased by 25%. Adding 3 cm of tissue thickness can require twice the input dose, and 8 cm of tissue can require 6 times the dose. Step angles further increase radiation doses. Strategies to reduce patient radiation exposure are shown in **Box 1**.

Box 1
Strategies to reduce patient radiation exposure

- Use radiation only when imaging is necessary to support clinical care
- Minimize use of cine
- Use stored fluoroscopy instead of cine when possible
- Minimize use of steep angles of x-ray beam
- Minimize use of magnification modes
- Minimize frame rate of fluoroscopy and cine
- Keep the image receptor close to the patient
- Use collimation to the fullest extent possible
- Monitor radiation dose in real time to assess patient risk-benefit during procedure
- Keep table as high as comfortably possible for the operator
- Vary imaging beam angle to minimize exposure to any single skin area
- Keep patient's extremities out of beam

IN-LABORATORY MONITORING OF GY

CTO PCI is a complex procedure in which the operator has much to consider. At our institution, the primary reason for terminating an unsuccessful procedure is the total Gy administered to the patient. Patients with obesity represent a subset in which radiation exposure is severely increased based on large tissue paths required for higher radiation input doses.

Therefore, in addition to ALARA, we measure total Gy every 30 minutes during the procedure, along with total contrast/MRCD and ACT. This 30-minute "time-out" makes the operator aware of key items that may result in changing strategies or procedure termination based on these factors. For example, if no progress has been made at 2 to 3 Gy, one may want to change strategies. Also, it reminds one to change imaging beam angles.

PROCEDURE TERMINATION

Criteria for procedure termination based on radiation exposure vary according local standards, and in coordination with a hospital-based radiation safety personnel, our program's policy follows. In general, if no significant progress has been achieved during CTO PCI, we terminate the procedure at 6 Gy. If the CTO has not been crossed with a guide wire by 8 Gy, we also terminate the procedure. If the case has not been completed by 12 Gy and the patient is not in a life-threatening state, eg, tamponade, the procedure is terminated.

PATIENT CARE POSTPROCEDURE RADIATION

All patients receiving greater than 5 Gy are identified in the catheterization laboratory at the end of the procedure and documented in the procedure notes and reports. Patient, family, and referring physicians are given an instructional handout on the signs and symptoms of radiation skin injury (**Fig. 2**). CTO PCI operator contact information is provided on the instructional handout if any radiation skin injury occurs or is suspected. Patients are instructed to avoid repeat radiation procedures for 2 to 3 months and longer if skin injury occurs.

REPEAT INVASIVE PROCEDURES IN PATIENTS WITH PREVIOUS HIGH RADIATION DOSES OR PRIOR SKIN INJURY

In general, patients receiving greater than 5 Gy without evidence of skin injury should NOT undergo elective repeat radiation exposure for 2 to 3 months. One must carefully examine the backs of these patients, as sometimes mild skin injury may go unnoticed. If no skin injury has occurred after 2 to 3 months and the risk/benefit ratio favors a successful procedure, one may elect to a repeat invasive procedure.

If a patient develops radiation skin injury, one should try to avoid future radiation exposure. This is particularly true for chronic ulceration. However, on occasion, these patients may present with unstable symptoms requiring invasive procedures. For those emergency procedures, one needs to avoid the previous area of skin injury. To accomplish this, we have devised a simple solution to radiologically identify and protect the site of prior skin injury.

RadPad (Worldwide Innovations and Technologies, Kansas City, KS, USA) is a sterile disposable radiation shield used over the access site to protect the operators from scatter. One can remove the sterile covering that covers this radiation shielding material. Then carefully measure the patient's healed radiation skin injury and exceed this measurement by one-half inch on each side. Next, using scissors, cut the radiation shield to these measurements. Then tape this radiation shield to the patient's back over the site of prior radiation injury. This will this allow the operator to easily fluoroscopically identify the area of previous skin injury and avoid this area during the procedure to prevent cumulative injury, as well as protect the prior area of radiation skin injury from new exposure.

VASCULAR ACCESS

Generally, the femoral artery is the preferred access site for the CTO PCI, although some prefer the radial approach, which is described in great detail in the article in this issue by Dr Stéphane Rinefret. Therefore, the discussion here is limited to femoral access. Bilateral femoral sheath placement before

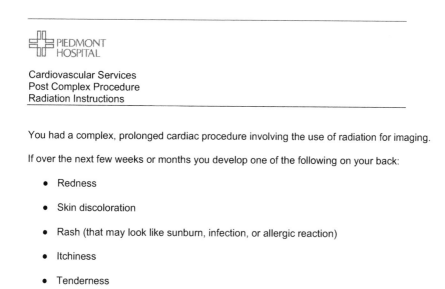

PIEDMONT HOSPITAL

Cardiovascular Services
Post Complex Procedure
Radiation Instructions

You had a complex, prolonged cardiac procedure involving the use of radiation for imaging.

If over the next few weeks or months you develop one of the following on your back:

- Redness

- Skin discoloration

- Rash (that may look like sunburn, infection, or allergic reaction)

- Itchiness

- Tenderness

- Drainage

Please contact immediately your physician who performed the procedure,   Dr.

_____ at the following number _____.

Fig. 2. Instructional handout on the signs and symptoms of radiation skin injury.

the administration of anticoagulation is mandatory in CTO PCI procedures. A 7-Fr or 8-Fr 45-cm sheath is placed for access to an antegrade approach. If a retrograde approach is likely, a second 7-Fr or 8-Fr 45-cm sheath is placed in the contralateral femoral artery. If it is certain that there is no retrograde option, one may place a 6-Fr sheath and the diagnostic catheter for contralateral injections. Even if the CTO vessel is seen to fill only by ipsilateral collaterals, it is important to place a 6-Fr sheath in the contralateral femoral, as the ipsilateral collaterals may disappear during the antegrade approach and previously unseen contralaterals may be recruited, which will be helpful for successful visualization of the distal vessel. Furthermore, contralateral filling of a CTO may have changed from the time of the diagnostic catheterization and one should at least quickly access with angiography if there is contralateral filling of the CTO vessel. On rare occasions, 3 arterial access sites are needed, eg, in patients after coronary artery bypass graft, in which the CTO vessel fills from 2 donor vessels.

GUIDE CATHETER SELECTION

In general, a 6-Fr to 8-Fr guiding catheter is placed for the antegrade approach, and if a simultaneous retrograde strategy is used, a second 90 cm guiding catheter is engaged in the collateral donor vessel. This will allow for seamless efficient transition between antegrade and retrograde intervention. In addition, having the retrograde catheter to be 90 cm will allow retrograde gear, such as a corsair, to be able to "reach" the antegrade guiding catheter.

Selection of the guiding catheter that supplies maximum support, good back-up, and low risk for aorta-ostial dissections is key to the success of all PCI procedures. Time spent on selecting a guiding catheter that will support you through the case is time well spent.

For left coronary arteries, extra back-up (EBU) is favored over Judkins curves; however, a Judkins curve may be preferred if it is an ostial or proximal LAD occlusion. We try to avoid side hole catheters for unprotected left coronary arteries, as they give one the false sense of no dampening but may cause ischemia from limiting blood flow. For the right coronary artery, Judkins right or Amplatz guide with or without side holes usually work well.

In summary, if a guide does not seat well, change as soon as possible, as a poorly seated guide will hamper you throughout the procedure. Alternative methods to augment guide catheter support include "mother-in-child" extensions, such as the guideliner and various balloon-anchoring techniques.

DUAL INJECTIONS

Based on thorough evaluation of the diagnostic angiogram and studying which projections will be the most helpful, pick the best RAO views and best LAD views and perform dual injections if there is evidence of contralateral filling.

CONCEPT OF CTO DAYS

CTO PCI is in general an elective procedure requiring significantly more contrast, radiation, patient risk, operator knowledge, and procedural time as compared with standard PCI. In addition, one should spend 20 to 30 minutes studying the diagnostic angiogram to plan the attack on the CTO, as well as alternative strategies if the primary strategy fails. Therefore, we do not recommend ad hoc CTO PCI but prefer elective planned CTO PCI. We favor the concept of "CTO days" in which 3 to 4 elective CTO PCI patients can be scheduled. In general, Mondays and Fridays are busy days in our laboratories and we have chosen Tuesdays and Thursdays as our CTO days. This allows the CTO operator to schedule his or her day accordingly, and not be constrained by time limits. Furthermore, 2 experienced CTO interventionists are scrubbed in per case, which we feel adds to the preprocedure assessment, procedural planning, and shifting strategies during the case as well as increasing CTO operator experience.

CTO OPERATOR TRAINING

CTO PCI is often referred to as the "last frontier" of interventional cardiology. Complex CTO PCI was initiated by a small group of interventionists in Japan some years ago, which slowly convinced interventionists in other parts of the world of the benefits of this procedure. Unfortunately, CTO PCI is still in its infancy stage and is being taught in ways that the inventor of angioplasty, Andreas Gruentzig, did so via conferences, workshops, and proctoring. Therefore, for an interventionalist interested in adopting CTO PCI techniques, one should attend dedicated CTO conferences, workshops, and internet-based programs in addition to learning through on-site proctoring. One should start with simple CTO PCI procedures, slowly progressing in lesion complexity. Also, try to scrub in with experienced CTO operators as often as possible, accept advice, and know when to quit.

STAFF TRAINING

Preprocedure, procedure, in-hospital postprocedure, and outpatient follow-up visits are essential for optimal patient outcomes for a successful

CTO PCI program. Members include registered nurses, physician assistants, and registered invasive cardiovascular specialists, all led by the CTO interventionist.

At the preprocedure outpatient visits, evaluate patient symptoms, perform noninvasive testing for ischemia and myocardial viability, and assess the ability of the patient to adhere to prolonged dual antiplatelet therapy, as well as initiate this therapy. Also, at the visit, assess for anemia and renal function, calculate GFR, holding potential nephrotoxic drugs, as well as metformin, and assess for recent extensive radiation exposure from prior cardiac procedures. Finally, assess the risk/benefit ratio of CTO revascularization and obtain informed consent from the patient.

Catheterization laboratory training of staff is paramount to a successful CTO program. At our institution, we have selected a finite number of staff to scrub in on CTO cases. We review the angiogram with the shift before the procedure so that everyone is one the same page during these complex procedures. As previously noted, our staff has a 30-minute timer that goes off throughout the CTO procedure to obtain an ACT, and advise the CTO operator on the total contrast used, MRCD, and cumulative Gy that the patient has received.

In-hospital postprocedure team members, including registered nurses, nurse practitioners, and physician assistants, are also extremely important for successful patient outcomes. The CTO operator needs to teach the hospital staff how to recognize signs and symptom complications that are seen with higher frequency with CTO PCI, such as hypotension from cardiac tamponade and increased risks of bleeding associated with bilateral large femoral sheaths. In addition, renal function after PCI needs to be assessed and instructions given on the resumption of medications that have been on hold. Reinforce to the patient the need for prolonged uninterrupted dual antiplatelet therapy. For patients given greater than 5 Gy, team members assist the CTO operator to instruct patient and family members what to look for if radiation injury occurs, as well as instructions to how to contact the CTO operator.

Outpatient follow-up visits should also reinforce the need for prolonged uninterpreted dual antiplatelet therapy and a careful examination of the patient's back for possible radiation-induced skin injury. If radiation skin injury is noted, the patient should be referred to the radiation specialist at your institution and told to avoid any future radiation exposure in the near-term future.

SUMMARY

CTO PCI in general is an elective procedure and involves a significant amount of preplanning, perhaps more so than any other coronary revascularization procedure. Attention to patient selection, appropriateness, technical strategy, risk factors, and operator experience are essential elements of CTO PCI revascularization success.

REFERENCES

1. Surber R, Schwarz G, Figulla HR, et al. Resting 12-lead electrocardiogram as a reliable predictor of functional recovery after recanalization of chronic total coronary occlusions. Clin Cardiol 2005;28(6):293–7.
2. Bonow RO. Identification of viable myocardium. Circulation 1996;94:2674–80.
3. Schelbert HR. The usefulness of positron emission tomography. Curr Probl Cardiol 1998;23:69–120.
4. Schwitter J, Wacker C, van Rossum A, et al. MRIM-PACT: comparison of perfusion-cardiac magnetic resonance with single-photon emission computed tomography for the detection of coronary artery disease in a multicentre, multivendor, randomized trial. Eur Heart J 2008;29:480–9.
5. Noguchi T, Miyazaki MD, Morii I, et al. Percutaneous transluminal coronary angioplasty of chronic total occlusions: determinants of primary success and long-term outcome. Catheter Cardiovasc Interv 2000;49:258–64.
6. Mollet NR, Hoye A, Lemos PA, et al. Value of preprocedure multislice computed tomography coronary angiography to predict the outcome of percutaneous recanalization of chronic total occlusion. Am J Cardiol 2005;95:240–3.
7. Aspelin P, Aubry P, Fransson SG, et al. Nephrotoxic effects in high-risk patients undergoing angiography. N Engl J Med 2003;348:491–9.
8. Mehran R, Aymong ED, Nikolsky E, et al. A simple risk score for prediction of contrast induced nephropathy after percutaneous coronary intervention. J Am Coll Cardiol 2004;44:1393–9.
9. Brosius FC 3rd, Hostetter TH, Kelepouris E, et al. Detection of chronic kidney disease in patients with or at increased risk of cardiovascular disease; a science advisory from the American Heart Association Kidney and Cardiovascular Disease Council; the Councils on High Blood Pressure Research, Cardiovascular Disease in the Young, and Epidemiology and Prevention; and the Quality of Care and Outcomes Research Interdisciplinary Working Group: developed in collaboration with the National Kidney Foundation. Circulation 2006;114:1083–7.
10. Barrett BJ, Carlisle EJ. Meta-analysis of the relative nephrotoxicity of high- and low-osmolality iodinated contrast media. Radiology 1993;188:171–8.

11. McCullough PA, Bertrand ME, Brinker JA, et al. Meta-analysis of the renal safety of isosmolar iodixanol compared with low-osmolar contrast media. J Am Coll Cardiol 2006;48:692–9.

12. Levine GN, Bates ER, Blankenship JC, et al. ACCF/AHA/SCAI guideline for percutaneous coronary intervention: a report of the American College of Cardiology Foundation/American Heart Association Task Force on Practice Guidelines and the Society for Cardiovascular Angiography and Interventions. J Am Coll Cardiol 2011;58:e44–122.

13. Freeman RV, O'Donnel M, Share T, et al. Nephropathy requiring dialysis after percutaneous coronary intervention and the critical role of an adjusted contrast dose. Am J Cardiol 2002;90:1068–73.

14. Hirshfeld JW Jr, Balter S, Brinker JA, et al. ACCF/AHA/HRS/SCAI clinical competence statement on physician knowledge to optimize patient safety and image quality in fluoroscopically guided invasive cardiovascular procedures: a report of the American College of Cardiology Foundation/American Heart Association/American College of Physicians Task Force on Clinical Competence and Training. J Am Coll Cardiol 2004;44:2259–82.

Wire Strategy as a First Option
Properties of the Tools

M. Nicholas Burke, MD

KEYWORDS

- Interventional guidewires • Chronic total occlusion • CTO PCI • Guidewire choices

KEY POINTS

- Chronic total occlusion percutaneous coronary intervention requires knowledge of guidewire characteristics.
- Different applications require specific types of wires with specific characteristics.
- Wire selection is determined by strategy, which is determined by anatomy.

INTRODUCTION

The successful completion of any percutaneous coronary intervention (PCI) is predicated on the successful placement of the distal aspect of a guidewire across a lesion while maintaining control of the proximal portion external to the patient. The guidewire is able to serve as a rail or track over which balloons, stents, and other interventional devices are advanced and deployed. Initial interventional procedures were done on a system where the wire was an integral part of the balloon such that the balloon and wire were fixed together, moving as a unit. This design did not allow for changing balloons or devices, without leaving the distal vessel unprotected when a new or different balloon or device was needed. The over-the-wire technique was subsequently developed which allowed the interventionalist to leave a wire in place, thus protecting the distal vessel while different interventional or diagnostic devices were used.[1,2]

The difficulty with chronic total occlusion (CTO) PCI is that advancing the guidewire successfully from the proximal vessel through the lesion into the distal true lumen is problematic. CTOs tend to be extremely hard and are often calcified.[3] Guidewires (if able to be advanced at all) would often end up in subintimal dissection planes or worse. Initial and even recent CTO PCI techniques focused on keeping the wire inside the true lumen

(so-called true to true) as it coursed through the CTO from the proximal to the distal vessel. Although the most straightforward and preferable, this strategy is often impossible to accomplish and has limited success rates.[4–7]

In order for CTO PCI to be more successful, novel strategies and techniques have been developed. These strategies and techniques often involve using the subintimal space intentionally (dissection-reentry technique) or approach the occlusion from both the proximal and distal portions of the vessel (retrograde technique, controlled antegrade and retrograde tracking [CART], reverse CART).[8] To facilitate these newer techniques and to improve the success rates for CTO PCI, guidewires have evolved with specific attributes that are used in specific fashions. It is the purpose of this article to discuss guidewire design and the differences in design as they apply to more modern CTO PCI techniques.

PERFORMANCE CHARACTERISTICS OF GUIDEWIRES

Guidewires, of course, come with a wide array of attributes, all of which affect their performance. Wires vary regarding their flexibility, trackability (ability to navigate tortuous anatomy), steering, and lubricity. They differ in their visibility (radiopacity), tendency to prolapse (likelihood of not following a branch takeoff despite the wire tip

Disclosures: The author is a consultant for BridgePoint Medical and Terumo Medical.
Minneapolis Heart Institute and Foundation, 920 East 28th Street, Minneapolis, MN 55407, USA
E-mail address: nburke@mplsheart.com

Intervent Cardiol Clin 1 (2012) 309–314
doi:10.1016/j.iccl.2012.03.004

interventional.theclinics.com

being positioned in the branch), degree of support (stiffness of the body of the wire), penetration power, and the degree of tactile feedback. Different attributes are more important in different situations and they also affect each other. For example, a wire may be lubricious, but this comes at the expense of tactile feedback to the operator, and a wire with good tactile feedback will generally be less slippery.

ANATOMY OF A GUIDEWIRE

1. The core: the main body of the wire that extends from the distal aspect up to or very near the absolute distal tip of the wire (**Fig. 1**)
2. The tip: the distal aspect of the wire
3. Coatings
4. Covers (also referred to as jackets or sleeves).

PROPERTIES OF GUIDEWIRES
The Core

Core material
The core is generally made up of a solid material that allows the transmission of torque from the operator's hands at the proximal end of the wire to the distal tip. Stainless steel has been the traditional material used. It is reasonably stiff, giving good torque transmission and support while being flexible to allow for good wire tracking. It is prone to bending or kinking, making the wire less durable. Nitinol (a nickel-titanium alloy) is a so-called shape-memory material, which resists permanent deformation despite being bent or misshapen. This resistance gives the wire the ability to be used repeatedly because it is not bent out of shape. Nitinol, however, is not as stiff as stainless steel and does not give as much support or torque transmission. High-tensile stainless steel is more kink resistant than regular stainless steel, so it retains its shape better and still provides good support and torque transmission.

Core taper
The core material is generally too stiff to safely pass down the coronary arteries and needs to be replaced by another less-traumatic material (**Fig. 2**). Rather than having an abrupt transition

to this material, which would substantially reduce the performance of the wire, the core tapers, becoming gradually covered by and transitioning into the tip material. The relative steepness of the taper affects the wire performance. A steeper or shorter taper provides more support and torqueability, whereas a gradual or longer taper allows for better wire tracking. The parabolic grind is a more novel taper or transition, which ostensibly allows for better support and torque transmission while still being trackable.

The Tip

Tip design
The tip stiffness is determined by the material that makes up the central aspect of the tip and how far the core extends into it (**Fig. 3**). In many wires, the core does not extend all the way to the end and is replaced by a shaping ribbon, which allows the tip to be easily bent into different angles. These tips tend to be softer and less traumatic to the vessel but are not as controllable. Alternatively, if the core extends all the way to the end, the tip tends to be stiffer with better torque transmission and subsequent steerability.

Tip coils
Most wires have spring coils wrapped around the distal aspect of the wire (**Fig. 4**). These coils allow for core transition and excellent tactile feedback. They also tend to improve radiopacity (visibility) and trackability depending on how long a segment of the wire is wrapped, but they can negatively affect the wire's ability to provide support.

Tip diameter
The tip diameter is also variable. Most coronary guidewires are 0.014″ throughout their length. Some wires have smaller tips allowing them to enter and traverse narrower channels, particularly the so-called microchannels (neovascular channels), which can develop inside a CTO.[3] The down side to this ability is that they are also more likely to enter tiny branch vessels or even exit the vessel entirely.

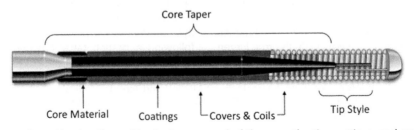

Fig. 1. Anatomy of a guidewire. The guidewire is composed of the core, the tip, coatings, and covers.

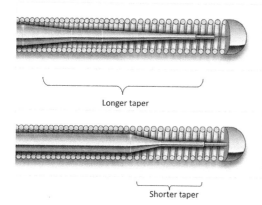

Fig. 2. Core taper. As the core approaches the tip, it tapers to be transitioned into other materials that are helpful for advancing or steering the guidewire. A longer taper results in a more trackable but less supportive wire, whereas a shorter taper results in the opposite effect.

Coatings

A coating is a microscopic layer that is often applied to wires to improve lubricity. There are 2 main types of coatings: hydrophilic and nonhydrophilic (hydrophobic). Hydrophilic coatings attract water. When in contact with water, they become a gel, which significantly decreases friction and increases trackability. Nonhydrophilic coatings repel water and do not require actuation. They also decrease friction and improve trackability but do so less than do hydrophilic coatings.

Covers, Jackets, or Sleeves

Covers are distinct from coatings, although the terms are often confused (**Fig. 5**). They are polymer or plastic that "jackets" the wire or covers it in a sleeve. Covers are hydrophilic, extremely lubricious, and provide smooth tracking through arteries. They reduce tactile feedback and because of their extreme slipperiness can enter and perforate small vessels if not used carefully. Nonjacketed wires most commonly have exposed coils at the tip, which reduce lubricity but improve tactile feedback.

Penetration Power

Penetration power is defined as the amount of force that a wire can exert on a given area or focal point (**Fig. 6**). This power is determined by the ratio of tip load (force required to buckle the wire tip when pushed against a hard surface) to the area over which this force is distributed. Penetration power is a more accurate way of assessing the ability of a guidewire to penetrate or pierce something than is tip stiffness, which is often reported by wire manufacturers. A wire's penetration power can be increased by increasing tip stiffness, decreasing tip area, or both.

GUIDEWIRE CHOICES FOR SPECIFIC TASKS IN CTO PCI

Not all CTOs are the same, and not all CTOs are approached in the same fashion. Anatomy dictates approach, which dictates guidewire choices. It is best to separate the tasks as follows: getting to the CTO (antegrade or retrograde), crossing the CTO (wire-escalation or dissection-reentry strategies, either antegrade or retrograde), and wire externalization.

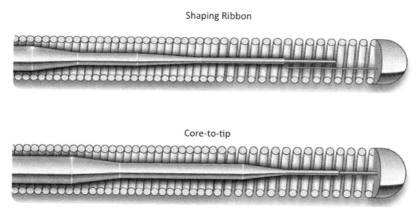

Fig. 3. Tip design. Guidewire tips can be of differing designs. The 2 most common designs feature either a tip-shaping ribbon or a core-to-tip design. The shaping ribbon is easily formed into a soft shape that is helpful for making turns or bends but is less steerable because of poorer torque transmission. In the core-to-tip design, the central core tapers but extends all the way to the end of the tip, resulting in a wire that is steerable but stiffer.

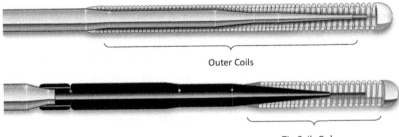

Outer Coils

Tip Coils Only

Fig. 4. Tip coils. Most guidewire tips have very thin wires wrapped around them forming a coil, which can affect tactile feedback, radiopacity (longer is more visible on radiograph), and wire support (longer coils tend to provide less support).

Getting to the CTO

Antegrade

Most proficient CTO operators use a workhorse wire to deliver whichever balloon or device they plan on working through to cross the CTO. This practice is done for 2 main reasons. First, the bend of the tip, which is often required to get to the CTO, is generally different from the bend used to cross a CTO. And second, the wires used to cross a CTO are either very lubricious or have high penetration power (or both) and are more likely to cause a dissection in the artery proximal to the CTO.

Retrograde

Most retrograde channels are small and can be extremely tortuous. To traverse this type of anatomy, a polymer-jacketed nontapered wire with low penetration power works best. In general, nontapered tips are used because of the increased chance of perforation with a smaller diameter tip. A tapered tip, however, is occasionally required to cannulate extremely small vessels.

Crossing the CTO

Wire-escalation strategy

The wire-escalation strategy is chosen when anatomy favors an attempt to advance the guidewire directly across the CTO from true lumen to true lumen (true-to-true), which can occur in either an antegrade or a retrograde direction. Historically, attempts were made with noncoated nontapered guidewires with increasing (escalating) tip stiffness designed to push or drill directly through the CTO. More recently, it has been found that a tapered-tip guidewire can often follow microchannels, which are present in many CTOs. In this case, the initial wire is a polymer-jacketed tapered-tip guidewire with low penetration force, which is used in an attempt to slide through the lesion. If this is unsuccessful, most modern CTO operators escalate directly to a jacketed tapered-tip guidewire with high penetration power.

Dissection-reentry strategy

The dissection-reentry strategy is chosen when the wire-escalation strategy seems likely to be unsuccessful or when the wire enters the subintimal space. This strategy can also be used in the antegrade or retrograde direction. This strategy has 2 distinct parts: dissection past the CTO and reentry from the false to the true lumen. In the dissection phase, after entering or presumably entering a dissection plane, a polymer-jacketed guidewire with low penetration power is used and the tip is prolapsed or "knuckled". This action results in an atraumatic leading edge, which is unlikely to perforate as it is advanced past the CTO. Occasionally, a stiffer polymer-jacketed wire is needed to develop sufficient force to pass through the subintimal space as it is knuckled. In

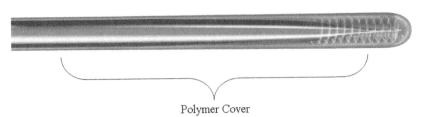

Polymer Cover

Fig. 5. Covers, jackets, or sleeves. Guidewires can be covered in a polymer or plastic that encases the inner structural wire elements. These covers are hydrophilic and highly lubricious but have limited tactile feedback.

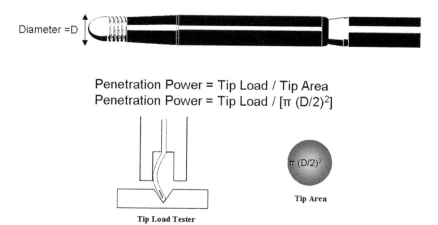

Penetration Power = Tip Load / Tip Area
Penetration Power = Tip Load / [π (D/2)^2]

Tip Load Tester

Tip Area

Fig. 6. The actual force exerted by the tip of the wire is referred to as the penetration power and is not the same as the tip stiffness. Penetration power is measured in force per unit area and subsequently is affected by both the tip stiffness and the diameter of the tip where the force is applied.

the reentry phase, it is necessary to penetrate into and then pierce the dissection flap to get access to the true lumen. In this case, a tapered jacketed guidewire with high penetration power is used.

Externalization

Wires used for externalization (only in retrograde cases) need to be as long as possible. The wire needs to pass antegrade up a guiding catheter, through the donor artery, collateral channel, CTO, vessel proximal to the CTO, and then retrograde down a guide, exiting the hemostatic valve with enough length left to control the wire and advance catheters, balloons, or stents on either end. Extending short guidewires is unadvisable for this purpose because of the possibility of kinking or separation. Standard 300-cm wires are difficult to use for externalization, particularly in taller patients. In general, a 330-cm or longer guidewire is preferable. The wire should be lubricious and kink resistant but not so supportive that it damages tortuous and fragile collateral channels.

TIP SHAPING

Virtually all guidewires used in CTO PCI come with straight tips because the tip shapes used in CTO PCI are distinctly different from those used in traditional PCI and are specific to their tasks. The bends used for the wire-escalation strategy and for collateral crossing are similar. In both cases, the lumen or area in which the tip rotates is narrow, so the bend is placed roughly 1 mm from the tip at an angle of approximately 20°. For the dissection-reentry strategy, the subintimal space is small, so the bend is also placed 1 mm from the tip. The

angle, however, is closer to 80° because the aim is to catch and pierce the dissection flap (**Fig. 7**).

SNARING

Although there are not wires that are used specifically for snaring and a discussion of snaring techniques is the subject of a separate article, a few comments here are appropriate. In general, it is best to use a large tulip snare in the ascending aorta to gently coax the retrograde wire into the guiding catheter so that it can be externalized. If the wire must be tightly grabbed, it is best to do

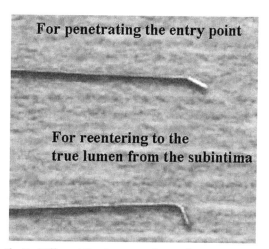

For penetrating the entry point

For reentering to the true lumen from the subintima

Fig. 7. Different tip shapes are better for various wire tasks. In general, all CTO bends should be short because the areas in which the wires are operating tend to be narrow. A straighter bend is best for penetrating and crossing a lesion, whereas a more acute bend is best for crossing from a dissection plane into the true lumen.

this on the tip. Two wires commonly used for externalization need special mention. The tip of the Rotawire (Boston Scientific, Nattick, MA, USA) can be broken if grasped too tightly. The Viperwire (CSI, Minneapolis, MN, USA) should not be folded over on itself on the body of the wire because it is then difficult to pull into the guide and advance.

SUMMARY

The techniques used in CTO PCI differ substantially from those used in more traditional coronary interventions. The equipment is also used differently, particularly guidewires. There are specific techniques for which guidewires with specific characteristics are used. Inappropriate guidewire choices are not only likely to result in unsuccessful procedures but can also be dangerous if used incorrectly. A clear understanding of these guidewires, their properties, and where they are best used is imperative for successful CTO PCI.

REFERENCES

1. Gruentzig A. Results from coronary angioplasty and implications for the future. Am Heart J 1982;103:779–83.
2. Levin DC, Ganz P, Friedman P, et al. Percutaneous transluminal coronary angioplasty with an over-the-wire-system. Radiology 1985;155(2):323–6.
3. Srivatsa SS, Edwards WD, Boos CM, et al. Histologic correlates of angiographic chronic total coronary artery occlusions: influence of occlusion duration on neovascular channel patterns and intimal plaque composition. J Am Coll Cardiol 1997;29:955–63.
4. Maiello L, Colombo A, Gianrossi R, et al. Coronary angioplasty of chronic occlusions: factors predictive of procedural success. Am Heart J 1992;124:581–4.
5. Ivanhoe RJ, Weintraub WS, Douglas JS Jr, et al. (King, Emory) Percutaneous transluminal coronary angioplasty for chronic total occlusions. Primary success, restenosis, and long-term clinical follow-up. Circulation 1995;85(1):106–15.
6. Stewart JT, Denne L, Bowker TJ, et al. Percutaneous transluminal coronary angioplasty in chronic coronary artery occlusions. J Am Coll Cardiol 1993;21(6):1371–6.
7. Tan KH, Sulke N, Taub NA, et al. Determinants of success of coronary angioplasty in patients with a chronic total occlusion: a multiple logistic regression model to improve selection of patients. Br Heart J 1993;70(2):126–31.
8. Surmely JF, Tsuchikane E, Katoh O, et al. New concept for CTO recanalization using controlled antegrade and retrograde subintimal tracking: the CART technique. J Invasive Cardiol 2006;18(7):334–8.

Antegrade Dissection and Reentry: Tools and Techniques

R. Michael Wyman, MD

KEYWORDS

- Chronic total occlusions • Percutaneous coronary intervention • Antegrade approach
- Dissection/reentry • BridgePoint device

KEY POINTS

- Antegrade dissection and reentry is an essential component of chronic total occlusion percutaneous coronary intervention.
- Previous techniques (STAR and its modifications) have been limited by low success rates and a lack of control over the site of reentry.
- The BridgePoint device was developed specifically for antegrade dissection and reentry and allows for efficient subintimal tracking and targeted reentry.
- Evolution of technique in conjunction with use of the BridgePoint device has resulted in an expansion of the anatomic subsets for which antegrade dissection and reentry can be successfully used.

INTRODUCTION

Coronary artery chronic total occlusions (CTO) remain the most challenging lesion subset for percutaneous intervention. Despite a growing body of evidence relating to poor long-term outcomes in patients with CTOs[1,2] and favorable effects of revascularization,[3,4] attempt rates in the United States remain low.[5] Reasons for this include historical perceptions related to low success rates and prolonged procedure times, and operator anxiety about working in the coronary subintimal space.

Multiple advances in technique and technology, many of them originally developed by Japanese operators, have led to significant improvements in procedural success.[6] Guidewire and microcatheter advances, and technique iterations, have refined the strategies of antegrade wire escalation, retrograde wiring, and retrograde dissection reentry to allow reproducible outcomes in the hands of highly skilled operators.[7] However, this experience has not lent itself to widespread adoption internationally for

three reasons: (1) the lack of a simplified and teachable strategy for how to approach any given anatomic situation; (2) the lack of emphasis on time (and radiation) efficiency; and (3) no previously available option for consistently successful antegrade dissection and reentry.

The hybrid approach to CTO percutaneous coronary intervention (PCI) was developed in response to these unmet needs.[8] An algorithm based on anatomic lesion characteristics defines the primary and subsequent secondary (tertiary and so forth) strategies (**Fig. 1**). The approach requires familiarity with all four potential options for wire crossing (**Fig. 2**), and just as importantly a willingness to move quickly and seamlessly from one strategy to another if failure modes are encountered. Antegrade dissection and reentry is as integral a component of wire crossing in the hybrid approach as any of the other three (antegrade wiring, retrograde wiring, retrograde dissection and reentry), yet it has suffered from inadequate tools to consistently achieve high levels of success. The lack of wire and catheter control over both ends of the CTO

Cardiovascular Interventional Research, Torrance Memorial Medical Center, 3445 Pacific Coast Highway, Suite 100, Torrance, CA 90505, USA
E-mail address: rmwcor@gmail.com

Intervent Cardiol Clin 1 (2012) 315–324
doi:10.1016/j.iccl.2012.04.001

interventional.theclinics.com

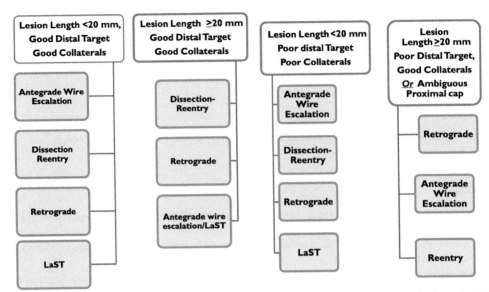

Fig. 1. The hybrid approach algorithm. Initial and subsequent strategies based on anatomic characteristics.

segment (as is available in retrograde dissection and reentry) has traditionally made successful reentry from the antegrade direction a challenge. The BridgePoint device (BridgePoint Medical, Plymouth, MN, USA), which is the only coronary CTO product to have been developed specifically for gaining reentry into the true lumen from the subintimal space, has now allowed antegrade

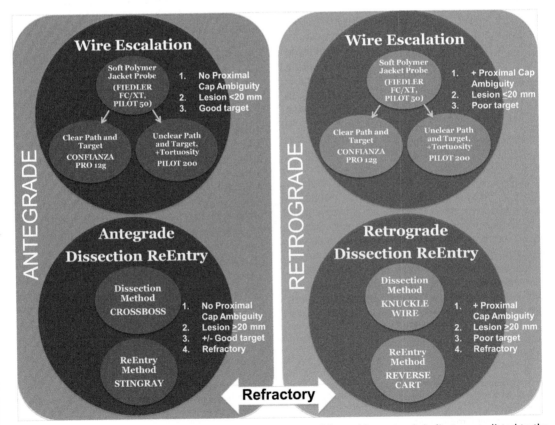

Fig. 2. The four crossing options for CTO intervention. Associated favorable anatomic indicators are listed to the right.

dissection and reentry to take it's appropriate place as an essential crossing option in the hybrid approach to CTO PCI.

ANATOMY

An important precept of the hybrid approach is that anatomic characteristics of the CTO dictate initial and subsequent strategy (see **Fig. 1**). A typical anatomic substrate that would lend itself to antegrade dissection and reentry as a primary strategy includes the following (**Fig. 3**):

- A well defined proximal cap
- Lesion length greater than 20 mm
- Moderate caliber distal vessel
- No large branches at the distal cap.

Other traditional indicators of CTO success, such as the presence of bridging collaterals, very long lesion length, tortuosity, and calcification, have little or no impact on the decision algorithm. In addition, as discussed later, a rapid evolution in technique has allowed for a significant expansion of the anatomic inclusion criteria for antegrade dissection reentry, such that an ambiguous proximal cap and diffusely diseased distal vessel become appropriate lesion subsets for primary attempts.

PREPROCEDURE PLANNING

As with any CTO intervention, meticulous preparation is a key to success. This includes physician, catheter laboratory, and patient-specific planning.

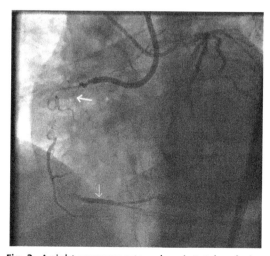

Fig. 3. A right coronary artery chronic total occlusion with favorable anatomic characteristics for primary antegrade dissection and reentry. The proximal cap (*thick arrow*) is well defined. The lesion length is greater than 20 mm. The distal vessel (*thin arrow*) reentry zone has an adequate caliber and there is no significant branch nearby.

The physician needs to be comfortable with the commonly used CTO skillsets (not limited to antegrade dissection and reentry), which include

- Advanced guide support techniques
- Specialized microcatheter (Tornus and Corsair; Asahi Intecc, Nagoya, Japan) manipulations
- Wire knuckling
- Wire puncturing techniques
- Balloon anchoring and trapping
- Contrast and radiation management.

The catheter laboratory should be well prepared in terms of equipment availability (preferably with the most frequently used CTO-specific gear on a separate "CTO cart") and a supportive and actively engaged staff.

Patient preparation includes detailed study of the diagnostic angiogram before proceeding, which obviates performing procedures in an ad hoc fashion. Careful attention should be paid to all of the aforementioned anatomic features and vessel take-off from the aorta, proximal tortuosity and disease, branches for anchoring, previously placed stents, donor vessel characteristics, collateral access, and so forth. Optimal imaging during the procedure is essential, which primarily necessitates the use of contralateral injections to visualize the distal vessel. Even in circumstances where ipsilateral collaterals are dominant and only faint contralateral collaterals are apparent, it is strongly recommended that dual access be obtained to prepare for the likely eventuality of loss of forward collateral visualization. This is particularly true for antegrade dissection and reentry, wherein antegrade contrast injections are strictly avoided to minimize enlargement of the subintimal space. Use of available state-of-the-art imaging equipment is also advisable, in terms of image quality and minimization of radiation dose.

PROCEDURAL APPROACH

Antegrade dissection reentry was originally described, in the coronary tree, as the subintimal tracking and reentry (STAR) technique.[9] As in peripheral (primarily superficial femoral artery [SFA]) CTO procedures, a knuckled wire is passed through and beyond the CTO segment, with distal true lumen access dependent on unpredictable and uncontrolled reentry, often into a small distal branch. Reconstruction of larger, more proximal branches, to preserve myocardial perfusion and enable adequate outflow (and thus proximal patency) can then be performed by "refenestration" techniques with polymer jacketed wires. Although an adequate angiographic result can be achieved, questions about true myocardial perfusion and long-term patency persist, and the authors themselves consider this to be a true bail-out, last chance technique, advising in addition against its use in the left anterior descending, where multiple sidebranches (ie, septal perforators) could be sheared off and not recovered.

Additional iterations of the STAR technique have been described, including contrast enhanced and mini-STAR,[10] yet these remain saddled with suboptimal control over the reentry site location, and relatively low rates of reentry success.

Despite these challenges, it has been clear for many years that any successful approach to CTO intervention requires the use of the subintimal space in a significant number of cases. The CTO experience in peripheral vessels, the Japanese operators' development of subintimal techniques for retrograde dissection and reentry (CART and reverse CART), and the failure of previous CTO niche devices that focused on true lumen crossing (eg, frontrunner, SafeCross) have all strongly reinforced this concept.

The BridgePoint device was specifically developed to take advantage of this frequent need for subintimal tracking to gain successful distal lumen access. There are three components to the system:

1. The CrossBoss catheter (**Fig. 4**): a multiple wire coiled shaft with a 0.014-in compatible through lumen, ending distally in a blunt, polished 1-mm distal tip. A proximal rotating device is rapidly spun outside the body by the operator, with gentle forward catheter pressure.

2. The Stingray balloon catheter (**Fig. 5**): an over-the-wire, 2.5-mm wide, flat balloon catheter that self-orients within the subintimal space. Two 180-degree opposed ports then allow controlled wire exit toward either the luminal space or the adventitial surface. Each port is located just proximal to a radiopaque marker.

3. The Stingray guidewire (see **Fig. 5**): a 12-g force wire with a shallow preformed angulated distal tip, and a 1-mm extruded segment that acts to catch tissue and penetrate through the subintima and into the true lumen.

A typical antegrade dissection reentry procedure with the BridgePoint device (**Fig. 6**) involves advancement of the CrossBoss catheter over a workhorse wire to the proximal cap, retraction of the wire into the catheter lumen, then rapid rotation of the catheter through the body of the CTO. The CrossBoss tracks into a distal true luminal position in 20% to 30% of cases,[11] but when the more frequent subintimal position is achieved, beyond the distal cap at an appropriate reentry position the guidewire is advanced and the catheter exchanged out for the Stingray balloon. This is brought into position over the guidewire and inflated to 3 to 4 atm. Visualization of the flat balloon is extremely important to enable orientation in

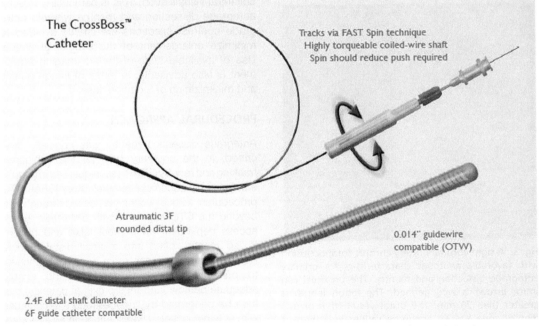

Fig. 4. The CrossBoss catheter. (*Courtesy of* BridgePoint Medical, Plymouth, MN; with permission.)

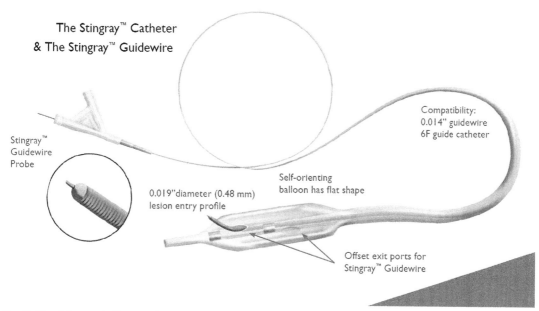

The Stingray™ Catheter
& The Stingray™ Guidewire

Stingray™
Guidewire
Probe

0.019"diameter (0.48 mm)
lesion entry profile

Self-orienting
balloon has flat shape

Compatibility:
0.014" guidewire
6F guide catheter

Offset exit ports for
Stingray™ Guidewire

Fig. 5. The Stingray balloon catheter and the Stingray wire. (*Courtesy of* BridgePoint Medical, Plymouth, MN; with permission.)

relation to the distal vessel lumen, and to determine the optimal view for reentry. This necessitates a meticulous preparation with 100% contrast. A contralateral angiogram is performed to demonstrate the balloon–vessel relationship, and the Stingray guidewire is then advanced and exited through the appropriate (luminal) port, with a direct puncture technique. A contralateral injection is again used to confirm the position of the wire in the lumen; the wire is rotated 180 degrees (away from the opposite wall) and advanced distally into the vessel. The Stingray balloon is then removed and an over-the-wire balloon or microcatheter is advanced, with subsequent exchange of the Stingray wire for a workhorse wire, over which all routine ballooning and stenting can then be performed.

Although the described technique is successful in many cases, extensive experience with the device by high-volume operators, and their collaboration on technique iteration, has led to multiple advances that have markedly influenced the anatomic opportunities for which the device is useful. These situations can be broadly grouped into overcoming difficulty with advancement of gear to the "base of operations" (ie, just beyond the distal cap for antegrade procedures) and overcoming challenges with reentry.

Gear Hangup

The proximal cap and body of the CTO are sometimes resistant to passage of the CrossBoss. In addition, an ambiguous or flush occluded proximal cap does not allow for entry of the CrossBoss into the CTO body. Finally, the CrossBoss can track into a side branch within the CTO segment, before arriving at the distal cap. These challenges can all be dealt with using similar techniques. For an ambiguous or resistant proximal cap, a stiff penetrating wire (either tapered tip hydrophilic or nontapered jacketed) is used to make initial progress over a very short distance (no more than 5–10 mm) using either the CrossBoss or another microcatheter as support. Longer traverses with the stiff wire, especially if followed by the support catheter, should be assiduously avoided because the potential for vessel perforation is enhanced. Instead, a knuckled wire (described in more detail later) is used to traverse most of the CTO segment, although not beyond the distal cap to the reentry site. The CrossBoss catheter is used to make the final subintimal dissection distally. This allows for a more refined dissection (with less enlargement of the space) while providing an adequate pathway for subsequent advancement of the Stingray catheter.

Reentry Challenges

These are represented by either loss of distal visualization of the reentry segment, usually by a compressive subintimal hematoma, or by a small diffusely diseased vessel beyond the distal cap. In the first case, preventive measures are a key: avoiding creation of a large subintimal space with antegrade injections, aggressive wire manipulation, or extended knuckling, and instead using the Crossboss catheter as detailed previously. If a hematoma forms, aspiration of the subintimal space with a separate

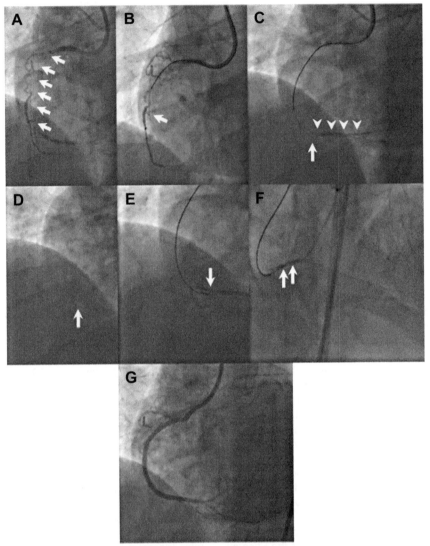

Fig. 6. Antegrade dissection reentry in a right coronary artery CTO (*A, arrows* denoting length of occlusion segment) using the BridgePoint device. The CrossBoss catheter is spun rapidly through the CTO (*B, C* with *arrow* at tip of crossboss and *arrowheads* at planned re-entry site) to a subintimal position just beyond the distal cap. The Stingray balloon (*D* with two radiopaque markers at *arrow*) is exchanged for and reentry is accomplished with the Stingray wire (*E, F,* with *arrows* showing wire puncture and reentry). After predilation and stenting, the vessel is recanalized (*G*). (*From* Whitlow PL, Burke MN, Lombardi WL, et al. Use of a novel crossing and re-entry system in coronary chronic total occlusions that have failed standard crossing techniques: results of the FAST-CTOs trial. JACC Cardiovasc Interv 2012;5:393–401.)

over-the-wire system can be attempted, although currently available over-the-wire balloons in the United States do not allow for simultaneous positioning with the Stingray in an 8Fr catheter guide.

In the case of a small and diffusely diseased distal vessel, a wire swap technique is very useful (**Fig. 7**): after initial puncturing into the lumen with the Stingray wire (which is not designed for finessed advancement through diseased vessels), the wire is removed and, with the Stingray balloon still inflated, swapped out for a jacketed wire. The latter

is then directed out the same exit port, allowing access into the lumen and manipulation into the distal vessel with enhanced success.

The Art of the Knuckle

A knuckled or looped wire has been used for many years in peripheral CTO intervention for rapid advancement through the subintimal space. This technique has now become an essential component of subintimal tracking in coronary CTO

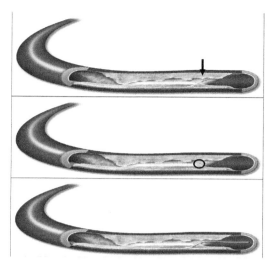

Fig. 7. The wire swap technique. An initial stick is made with the Stingray wire through the distal port of the Stingray catheter (*top*), from the subintimal space and into the lumen. The disease beyond the distal cap limits further advancement of the wire and it is removed (*middle*) with the balloon position maintained. A polymer jacketed wire is advanced and accesses the same exit port (*bottom*) with easier manipulation into the distal vessel. (*Courtesy of BridgePoint Medical, Plymouth, MN; with permission.*)

PCI for antegrade and retrograde approaches. A knuckled wire has the advantage of quickly and safely traversing occlusive anatomy, particularly in those situations where the course of the vessel is not well understood. In comparison, use of stiff, tapered tip wires to cover the same geography can be time consuming and prone to perforation. This is because the adventitia, although very distensible in response to blunt force delivered over a large surface area (ie, the knuckle wire), can be punctured easily with a penetrating force delivered at a single focus (ie, a stiff tapered tip wire).

The most frequently used wires for knuckling in the coronary tree are polymer jacketed wires, either soft (with or without a tapered tip) or stiff and nontapered. The goal is to catch the tip of the wire (whether or not it has been preshaped into the classic "umbrella handle") on tissue within the vessel architecture, so that a loop is formed in a more proximal segment of the wire as it is advanced. This working aspect of the knuckle is often at the junction between the radiopaque coils and the stiffer more radiolucent part of the wire (**Fig. 8**). At times, depending on vessel tortuosity and calcification, the amount of force necessary to advance the knuckle can be significant. This sensation runs counter to even the most experienced interventionalists' concept of wire advancement through the coronary tree. However, as long as

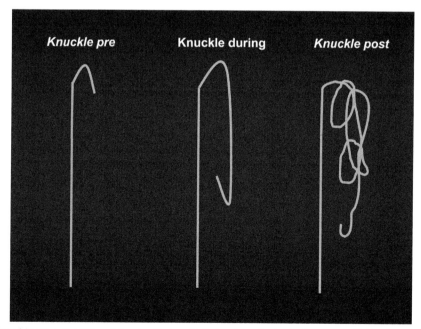

Fig. 8. The knuckle wire. Traditional "umbrella handle" shaping of wire before entry (*left*). The working loop of the knuckle (*middle*) is more proximal, often at the junction of the soft and stiffer segments. After removal, the wire is frequently quite deformed (*right*).

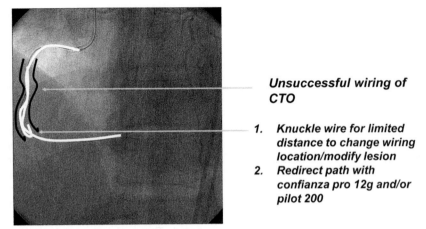

Unsuccessful wiring of CTO

1. *Knuckle wire for limited distance to change wiring location/modify lesion*
2. *Redirect path with confianza pro 12g and/or pilot 200*

Fig. 9. Limited antegrade subintimal tracking.

the size of the loop is controlled, such that it is not significantly larger than the perceived diameter of the vessel, this forward force remains safe and time efficient. Loop size management depends on the type of wire used (soft jacketed wires tending to form smaller loops) and on the relationship between the support catheter and the knuckle. If the loop becomes too large, advancement of the support catheter and retraction of the wire (at times completely back into the catheter) with subsequent reknuckling often controls loop size.

Additional advantages of knuckling include its ability to bypass areas of resistance met by more focused catheters (as discussed previously in relation to CrossBoss techniques), and its tendency to avoid entry into sidebranches that are a smaller diameter than the main vessel.

Limited Antegrade Subintimal Tracking and Redirection

A more recently described antegrade dissection reentry technique,[12] limited antegrade subintimal tracking and redirection (LAST) involves the advancement of a knuckled wire down to, but not beyond (as in STAR), the distal cap. A support catheter is then brought to the same position and a stiff wire (either polymer jacketed, nontapered, or nonjacketed and tapered), usually with a more exaggerated tip bend, is used to try and reenter the distal true lumen (**Fig. 9**). Theoretically, the wire should engage the tissue in the distal body of the CTO to gain luminal entry, rather than attempting a true reentry from the subintimal space beyond the distal cap. This technique, as noted

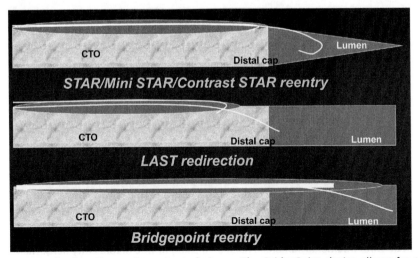

Fig. 10. Three antegrade dissection and reentry techniques. The BridgePoint device allows for the only true control over reentry.

Table 1
Technical success and MACE in the FAST-CTO trial compared with other CTO device trials

	FAST-CTOs	Crosser	SafeCross	Frontrunner
No. of patients	147	125	116	107
Technical success	77%	61%	54%	56%
30-d MACE	4.8%	8.8%	6.9%	8%

by its acronym, is also a final bailout option should all other strategies fail, but one that has advantages over STAR and has met with fairly good anecdotal success.

Fig. 10 is a schematic depiction comparing the various antegrade dissection and reentry techniques. LAST has more potential control over the site of reentry than STAR, but neither has the predictable and accurate control of BridgePoint nor the same level of success.

CLINICAL RESULTS

A number of published reports have delineated the worldwide experience with the BridgePoint device, from first-in-man descriptions[13] to European and isolated case reports.[14,15] The most comprehensive data come from the recently published outcomes of the US Facilitated Antegrade Steering Technique in Chronic Total Occlusions (FAST-CTO) trial.[11] A total of 150 refractory CTOs, defined as either a failed attempt within the last year or failed wiring attempts during the index procedure, were treated with the device. The primary end point was successful placement of a guidewire within the distal true lumen, with secondary end points of fluoroscopy and procedure time. The safety end point was major adverse cardiac event (MACE) out to 30 days. Anatomic exclusion criteria included saphenous vein graft,

in-stent, or aorto-ostial lesions, and a small distal vessel caliber (<1.5 mm) or large branch at the distal cap. There was no exclusion for lesion length, which by Core lab QCA measurement was 22 mm, similar to most other CTO device and registry studies.

Technical success results compared with the historical control of previous CTO device trials are shown in **Table 1**. The success rate of 77% compared favorably and led to Food and Drug Administration approval. Equally important, there was a definite learning curve noted (**Fig. 11**), with success rates in the latter half of the trial population increasing to 86%. Insofar as many of the investigators had no prior experience with the device, familiarity clearly led to content.

Fluoroscopy and procedure time were 105 and 44 minutes, significantly less than the historical controls. Thirty-day MACE was 4.8%, with two late deaths (>16 days) unrelated to the procedure and five device-related perforations (3.4%), none of which required pericardiocentesis or surgery.

SUMMARY

Percutaneous intervention on CTOs in the coronary tree, although often clinically indicated, has been inhibited because of the perception of low success rates; long procedure times; high radiation exposure; and safety concerns, particularly in regards to operator comfort levels with working in the subintimal space. With the development of an objective and teachable strategy for approaching CTO intervention safely and efficiently (the hybrid approach), many of these concerns can be alleviated. Antegrade dissection and reentry is an essential component of the hybrid approach, largely because of the availability of the Bridge-Point device. Initial experience with this device, and subsequent rapid evolution of technique, has led to a progressive expansion of the anatomic subsets for which the device can allow successful recanalization of these difficult lesions.

REFERENCES

1. Hannan EL, Wu C, Walford G, et al. Incomplete revascularization in the era of drug eluting stents: impact

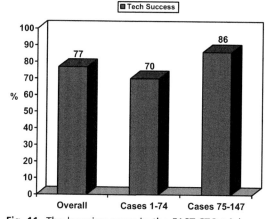

Fig. 11. The learning curve in the FAST-CTO trial.

on adverse outcomes. JACC Cardiovasc Interv 2009; 2:17–25.

2. Claessen BE, van der Schaaf RJ, Verouden NJ, et al. Evaluation of the effect of a concurrent chronic total occlusion on long term mortality and left ventricular function in patients after primary percutaneous intervention. JACC Cardiovasc Interv 2009;2:1128–34.

3. Kirschbaum SW, Baks T, van den Ent M, et al. Evaluation of left ventricular function 3 years after percutaneous coronary intervention of chronic total occlusions. Am J Cardiol 2008;101:179–85.

4. Joyal D, Afilaol J, Rinfret S. Effectiveness of recanalization of chronic total occlusions: a systematic review and meta-analysis. Am Heart J 2011;160: 179–87.

5. Grantham JA, Marso SP, Spertus J, et al. Chronic total occlusion angioplasty in the United States. JACC Cardiovasc Interv 2009;2:479–86.

6. Sumitsuji S, Inoue K, Ochiai M, et al. Fundamental wire technique and current standard strategy of percutaneous intervention for chronic total occlusions with histopathologic insights. JACC Cardiovasc Interv 2011;4:941–51.

7. Morino Y, Kimura T, Hayashi Y, et al, J-CTO Registry Investigators. In-hospital outcomes of contemporary percutaneous coronary intervention in patients with chronic total occlusions: insights from the J-CTO registry (multicenter CTO registry in Japan). JACC Cardiovasc Interv 2010;3:143–51.

8. Brilakis ES, Grantham JA, Rinfret S, et al. A percutaneous treatment algorithm for crossing coronary chronic total occlusions. JACC Cardiovasc Interv 2012;5:367–79.

9. Colombo A, Mikhail GW, Michev I, et al. Treating chronic total occlusions using subintimal tracking and reentry: the STAR technique. Catheter Cardiovasc Interv 2005;64:407–11.

10. Carlino M, Godino C, Latib A, et al. Subintimal tracking and re-entry technique with contrast guidance: a safer approach. Catheter Cardiovasc Interv 2008;72:790–6.

11. Whitlow PL, Burke MN, Lombardi WL, et al. Use of a novel crossing and re-entry system in coronary chronic total occlusions that have failed standard crossing techniques: results of the FAST-CTOs trial. JACC Cardiovasc Interv 2012;5:393–401.

12. Lombardi WL. Retrograde PCI: what will they think of next? J Invasive Cardiol 2009;21:543.

13. Whitlow PL, Lombardi WL, Arraya M, et al. Initial experience with a dedicated coronary re-entry device for revascularization of chronic total occlusions. Catheter Cardiovasc Interv 2011. [Epub ahead of print].

14. Werner GS, Schofer J, Sievert H, et al. Multicentre experience with the BridgePoint devices to facilitate recanalization of chronic total coronary occlusions through controlled subintimal re-entry. EuroIntervention 2011;7:192–200.

15. Brilakis ES, Lombardi WL, Banerjee S. Use of the Stingray guidewire and the Venture catheter for crossing flush coronary chronic total occlusions due to in-stent restenosis. Catheter Cardiovasc Interv 2010;76:391–4.

Retrograde Procedural Planning, Skills Development, and How to Set Up a Base of Operations

James C. Spratt, MD, FRCP, FESC[a],*,
Julian W. Strange, MBChB, MD, FRCP[b]

KEYWORDS

- Chronic total occlusion • Retrograde access • Angiography • Skills development

KEY POINTS

- Retrograde access has improved procedural success in the treatment of chronic total occlusions (CTOs), but it requires a thorough understanding of the principles involved and careful planning.
- Retrograde access may be preferable in situations of predictable antegrade complexity or in situations where retrograde access is technically easier.
- Training to become a skilled retrograde operator should include background reading, attendance at training conferences, and performing cases under the supervision of an experienced proctor.
- Angiographic assessment is the bedrock of procedure planning.

 Videos of Proximal anatomic ambiguity; Ostial occlusions; and A distal CTO cap at a major bifurcation accompany this article.

INTRODUCTION
Background and Historical Perspective

Chronic total occlusions (CTOs) represent a commonly occurring lesion subset, historically associated with lower procedural success rates of revascularization, both percutaneously and by coronary artery bypass grafting (CABG).[1] Several recent developments in techniques have been associated with improved procedural success when adopted on a local basis. Of these, access via donor collaterals to the CTO segment (retrograde access) was first described in 1990,[2] and when more widely adopted and refined has been associated with improvements in procedural success.[3] Despite this, it is unclear how widely retrograde access has been adopted. Data from the EuroCTO registry suggest that the retrograde procedure is used in approximately 15% of CTO procedures.[4] Given that these data represent a subset of CTO specialists, it would seem likely that retrograde access represents only a small minority of the techniques currently used to treat CTOs.

It is probable that there are several factors influencing this failure of uptake, including: unfamiliarity with the technique; lack of an educational framework within which the technique is delivered; and lack of clarity as to when and how to apply the technique. Some of these issues are addressed further in this article.

Skills Development

Although this article describes a step-by-step approach to the retrograde procedure, it is not a substitute for hands-on training. It is important,

[a] Department of Cardiology, Forth Valley Royal Hospital, Stirling Road, Larbert FK5 4WR, UK; [b] Bristol Heart Institute, University Hospitals Bristol NHS Foundation Trust, Level 5, Bristol Royal Infirmary, Marlborough Street, BS1 3NU, Bristol, UK
* Corresponding author.
E-mail address: james.spratt@nhs.net

Intervent Cardiol Clin 1 (2012) 325–338
doi:10.1016/j.iccl.2012.05.001

interventional.theclinics.com

however, to support the technical proficiency required for the retrograde procedure with a fundamental understanding of the underlying principles. It is the authors' belief that the training required to become a skilled retrograde operator is multifaceted and should include background reading, attendance at training conferences, and performing cases under the supervision of an experienced proctor. The intricacies of the procedure are such that it is not recommended for operators to attempt their first procedure unsupervised. Abbreviations used in this article are listed in **Box 1**.

Physiologic and Histopathologic Rationale

CTO lesions are made up of proximal and distal fibrous caps, which encase a softer core of organized thrombus and lipid. There has been some suggestion from pathologic data that the formation of the CTO cap is dependent on the pressures it is exposed to.[5] The proximal CTO cap is typically exposed to higher pressures (diastolic = 60–80 mm Hg) and therefore tends to form a less benign or blunt cap (**Fig. 1**). The distal cap, however, is exposed to lower pressures and as a consequence may be softer, more tapered, and hence easier to

penetrate. Histopathologic comparisons of proximal and distal caps reveal the former to be thicker, with more dense collagen-rich fibrous tissue.[6]

PROCEDURE PLANNING: CASE SELECTION
When Retrograde Access May be Preferable

Retrograde access may be preferable in situations of predictable antegrade complexity or situations whereby retrograde access is technically easier. It is partly for this reason that the adoption of retrograde skills leads to improved procedural success. These situations are often not binary and represent a continuum wherein the threshold for retrograde access will be lower with greater experience.

Anatomic subsets of predictable antegrade complexity are shown in **Fig. 2**.

Proximal Anatomic Ambiguity

Proximal anatomic ambiguity is illustrated in Video 1 (available online at http://www.interventional.theclinics.com/). If the location/nature of the proximal cap cannot be defined, this significantly limits the ability to escalate penetration force. Although there are occasions when the proximal cap can be defined further with adjunctive imaging techniques (intravascular ultrasonography [IVUS] coronary computed tomographic angiography [CTA]), there are limitations to the applicability of these techniques. IVUS requires the presence of a side branch large enough to accommodate an IVUS catheter at, or very near, the proximal cap. CTA can help to define and localize the proximal cap, but in the absence of highly accurate coregistration this can be of limited applicability.

In these situations retrograde access may be preferable, either from a primary procedural success perspective or by the presence of a retrograde wire/microcatheter to help define the proximal cap (**Fig. 3**) and enable escalation of therapy.

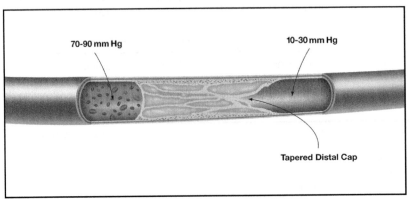

70-90 mm Hg   10-30 mm Hg

Tapered Distal Cap

Fig. 1. Higher perfusion pressures lead to a harder, blunter, less "favourable" proximal cap of the CTO.

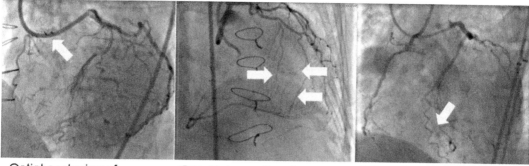

| Ostial occlusion of RCA | Good interventional collaterals | Bifurcation at distal cap of CTO |

Fig. 2. Subsets favouring a primary retrograde approach are shown.

Ostial Occlusions

An ostial occlusion is illustrated in Video 2 (available online at http://www.interventional.theclinics.com/). True ostial occlusions are complex from an antegrade approach for several reasons, including lack of guide support, and anatomic ambiguity and angulation: issues that may be better addressed retrogradely.

- True ostial occlusions are inevitably associated with reduced guide support and increased movement of the guide, making proximal cap puncture very challenging.
- Ostial occlusions (of left main stem [LMS] and right coronary artery [RCA]) are commonly associated with aortic wall fibrocalcification, increasing the requirement for high penetration forces.
- Ostial occlusions often contain either a significant degree of angulation or anatomic ambiguity, which can be minimized or negated by a primary retrograde approach.

Distal CTO Cap at a Major Bifurcation

A distal CTO cap at a major bifurcation is illustrated in Video 3 (available online at http://www.interventional.theclinics.com/). Antegrade recanalization is associated with subintimal entry in up to 45% of cases,[5] and the risk of this subintimal passage increases with the length of the CTO. Hence, the combination of a long (>20 mm) CTO with a distal cap at a major bifurcation results in the risk of losing a major side branch. This risk is minimized by retrograde access. An increased angulation at a distal cap bifurcation also increases the risk of subintimal entry at the bifurcation. If the reentry to the true lumen is distal to the bifurcation, the risks of major side-branch loss are high.

Small or Diseased Distal Vessel

A small diseased distal vessel will complicate all antegrade approaches: the risks of subintimal access are high with any CTO longer than 20 mm, and current methods of true lumen reentry

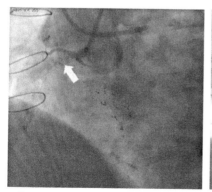

Proximal Cap Ambiguity

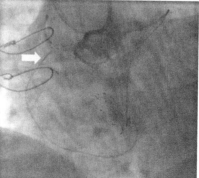

Proximal Cap Anatomy Clarified by Retrograde Corsair Position

Fig. 3. The role of a retrograde approach in clarifying proximal anatomic ambiguity is demonstrated: advancing retrograde equipment to the level of the proximal cap provides information on its location.

(parallel wire; see-saw; IVUS-guided reentry; Stingray [BridgePoint Medical Systems, Minneapolis, MN, USA]) require good visualization and filling of the distal vessel. With all of these methods, the difficulty of reentry increases with the decreasing size of true lumen.

Anatomic Subsets of Retrograde Preference

Good interventional collaterals

Predictable, safe, and easily achieved retrograde access may suggest a primary retrograde approach, particularly when combined with one of the anatomic subsets already described. In the majority of cases this will mean septal access, given the reduced risk of collateral related complications encountered via this route; however, this is also critically dependent on operator experience. On an early part of the operator's learning curve it is preferable to attempt cases for which retrograde access is more predictable.

PROCEDURE PLANNING: GENERAL ISSUES

- *Anticoagulation.* Retrograde procedures are associated with a higher risk of thrombotic complications caused by several factors, including longer length of procedure, long periods of relative arterial stasis (especially in occluded arteries with proximal anchoring balloons), and the increased use of adjunctive equipment. It is therefore recommended that unfractionated heparin is given in a weight-adjusted dose to achieve an activated clotting time (ACT) of more than 350 seconds. The ACT should be checked every 30 minutes and further heparin given if required. The use of glycoprotein IIb/IIIa receptor antagonists is not recommended because of the relatively high incidence of microperforations, which in the absence of excessive anticoagulation are usually not clinically significant.
- *Radiation.* It is important to minimize radiation exposure while maintaining procedural efficiency and safety. Simple measures to achieve this include reducing the frame rate, minimizing acquisition sequences, rotating the camera through different angles, and keeping an individualized patient radiation record.
- *Contrast.* The risk of contrast nephropathy increases with increasing contrast load. Contrast should therefore be used parsimoniously. Indeed, there are specific reasons why a retrograde procedure should need less contrast. The position of the retrograde equipment provides constant visualization, otherwise provided by contrast. Moreover, antegrade injection of contrast is very unlikely to be helpful and may cause hydraulic dissection of the proximal vessel, increasing the need for subsequent stenting and reducing distal visualization because of intravascular hematoma. Indeed a case can be made for covering the antegrade guide until required for stent/balloon delivery.
- *Access sites.* In general this is determined by the French-unit size required. While there are some advantages to larger French sizes (allow "trapping" balloons [**Fig. 4**]) that permit the use of balloon anchors and supportive microcatheters such as the Tornus (Asahi Intecc, Nagoya, Japan), it is possible to perform retrograde procedures via a 6F approach. As dual-access sites are mandatory, defaulting to the right radial and right femoral may be preferable to a bi-femoral approach. For additional support and to reduce any adverse effect of peripheral tortuosity, long (>45 cm) sheaths are recommended.
- *Catheter selection.* It is advisable to use supportive guides, preferably with larger French sizes as already discussed. For accessing the donor vessel, a short (90 cm) guide is preferred (especially when using epicardial collaterals), which can be made by shortening the guide and reconnecting with the sheath 1 French smaller. Side-hole catheters are recommended for the RCA (to reduce the risk of hydraulic dissection), but not the LMS, where it is critically important to recognize early damping (and potential dissection risk).

PROCEDURE PLANNING: ANGIOGRAPHIC ASSESSMENT

Angiographic assessment is the bedrock of procedure planning. The angiogram should be assessed according to specific criteria (**Fig. 5**) to help plan procedural strategy. Although optimal angiographic planning requires dual injections from both left and right coronary ostia, this is seldom available from referring non-CTO operators and is thus a necessary prerequisite before starting a CTO procedure. Several additional caveats are an important requirement for adequate angiographic images:

- Careful analysis of collateral filling requires virtual absence of camera panning as well as consideration of collateral filling in several projections.

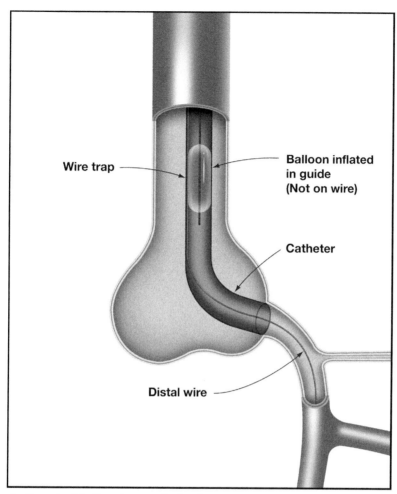

Wire trap

Balloon inflated in guide (Not on wire)

Catheter

Distal wire

Fig. 4. The use of a "trapping" balloon is a standard technique in CTO angioplasty which facilitates exchange of over-the-wire equipment. A balloon is placed in the guide (not on a wire) and inflated, thereby fixing the distal wire enabling removal and delivery of over-the-wire equipment.

- A wide field of view and potential reduction in camera magnification is usually required to appreciate the direction of collateral filling and to avoid missing the course of "wandering" collaterals.

Long runs are required to properly assess CTO length (although this still may be overestimated without dual injections). Reconstruction of the anatomy can be especially challenging after CABG, and may require simultaneous injection with more than 2 catheters and careful reconstruction of a good-quality CTA image.

As many CTO cases are referred by non-CTO operators, it is probable that images may not meet all the aforementioned criteria, making traditional analysis of collateral supply challenging. In such cases the authors have investigated the utility of applying an image analysis algorithm (**Fig. 6**).

Within the context of angiographic analysis, the following specific areas should be carefully analyzed.

Degree of Coronary Disease

Is there single-, 2-, or 3-vessel coronary disease? What order of revascularization is planned? Although there is no evidence-based answer to inform whether donor vessel disease should be treated before or after the CTO vessel, the following considerations may apply.

Considerations favoring pretreatment of donor disease

Does donor vessel disease limit the collateral supply and therefore the visualization of the vessel?

Would pretreatment of donor vessel disease improve the safety of the CTO procedure?

Chronic Total Occlusion Algorithm

1. With a dual injection:

Look for these features:
Ambiguous proximal cap
Poor distal target
Appropriate collaterals
Significant side branches

2. If 'yes' to above features:

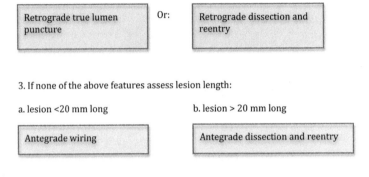

| Retrograde true lumen puncture | Or: | Retrograde dissection and reentry |

3. If none of the above features assess lesion length:

a. lesion <20 mm long

Antegrade wiring

b. lesion > 20 mm long

Antegrade dissection and reentry

4. If failure to progress with initial technique, change of strategy:

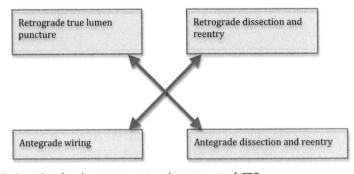

| Retrograde true lumen puncture | Retrograde dissection and reentry |

| Antegrade wiring | Antegrade dissection and reentry |

Fig. 5. A suggested algorithm for the assessment and treatment of CTOs.

Would instrumentation of a diseased donor vessel increase the risk of adverse cardiovascular events?

Considerations favoring initial treatment of the CTO

Would percutaneous treatment of the donor vessel limit the ability to treat the CTO? (eg, by covering a collateral with a stent.)

Would pretreatment of donor vessel disease preclude future surgical options? This consideration may depend on which artery is the CTO. For example, an occluded left anterior descending (LAD) coronary artery may argue for a lower threshold for CABG, whereas the poor 1-year patency[7] of saphenous vein graft to RCA or circumflex (Cx) may argue for a more aggressive percutaneous approach.

Nature of the Proximal Cap/Distal Cap

The same angiographic consideration should be given to both proximal and distal caps of the CTO.

Can the proximal cap of the CTO be defined or is it anatomically ambiguous (it is rarer for the distal cap to be anatomically ambiguous)? Is it tapered or blunt in nature? (see **Fig. 1.**) What is its relationship to proximal anatomy: is it a bifurcation of a major side branch?

Length of CTO Segment

Increasing the length of the CTO segment is no longer a limiter for procedural success, but does determine procedural strategy. It is safer and more efficacious to traverse long CTO segments by the use of a knuckle wire (**Fig. 7**), via both antegrade and retrograde procedures. A knuckle wire is created when a soft wire (such as the Fielder XT; Asahi Intecc) or polymer-coated wire (such as the Pilot 200; Abbot Vascular, Baltimore, MD, USA) is pushed against tip resistance so that it folds over, forming a knuckle. A microcatheter is kept close to the distal end of the knuckle to help provide sufficient support and minimize the knuckle size. The knuckled wire helps to negate the effect of anatomic ambiguity within the CTO segment, most commonly found in the form of tortuosity. A knuckle wire is also an effective way to apply significant force to negotiate a highly resistant occluded segment while minimizing the risk of perforation.

Tortuosity

Tortuosity remains an important limiter of procedural success, primarily for 2 reasons:

1. Increased tortuosity equates to increased lesion resistance caused by loss of coaxial pushing force, thereby increasing the need for higher levels of supportive interventional equipment (or adjunctive support techniques such as balloon anchors). When combined with high inherent lesion resistance (eg, in the presence of highly calcified lesions), this may limit procedural success.
2. Tortuosity is associated with higher levels of anatomic ambiguity. The effects of this can be minimized by the use of a knuckle wire.

Calcification

Calcification is commonly associated with CTOs of long duration and especially in post-CABG patients. Its presence, as with tortuosity, is an important predictor of procedural failure and should inform procedural technique. In the particular context of a retrograde procedure, calcification indicates the need for a highly supportive interventional setup and may also indicate the need for adjunctive interventional strategies such as rotational atherectomy.

PROCEDURE PLANNING: COLLATERAL ASSESSMENT

When assessing collaterals the most commonly used system is the Werner classification,[8] in which collateral channels (cc) are divided up into the following:

- cc 0: invisible/near invisible connections
- cc 1: small spidery connections
- cc 2: epicardial-like connections.

Collaterals can be further divided into 2 basic categories—epicardial and septal collaterals—and have specific crossing profiles, indicating they should be assessed separately.

Collateral Dominance

Particularly when assessing the collateral supply of the RCA, it is often evident that one collateral system (either Cx–posterior left ventricular [PLV] branch or LAD–posterior descending branch [PDA] of the RCA) is dominant: that is, it fills preferentially by that system. The dominance of the collateral system may be assessed by the direction of the filling of the distal bed, and may have important implications on crossability and tolerability. The concept of collateral dominance may also be applied to a very large (often epicardial) collateral. If this is used as an interventional collateral, it may result in significant ischemia, and if damaged may result in myocardial damage.

Septal Versus Epicardial Collaterals

In general, retrograde access via septal collaterals is safer than the epicardial equivalents, and should be preferred in most cases until experience has been accumulated with standard retrograde techniques. A possible exception to this rule is the presence of relatively straight epicardial collaterals in patients after CABG; in this situation pericardial tamponade is unlikely.

SEPTAL COLLATERALS

There is considerable variation in septal anatomy, but in general very proximal septal channels (from the LAD) connect rarely to the RCA and to the PLV branch of the RCA if they do, whereas all distal septal channels communicate to the posterior descending branch (PDA) of the RCA (**Fig. 8**). These channels are best appreciated in a combination of cranial (right anterior oblique [RAO]/anteroposterior) and straight RAO projections.

4 Key Stages for Retrograde Planning & Collateral Analysis

1 Angiographic Review

Review all angiographic films.

Select 3 to 4 films to further analyse.

RAO 30 & RAO cranial views.

Collaterals that are optimised with contrast. Frame 50 shown.

2 Collateral Analysis

Select the frames with contrast that reaches the CTO, or where collateral connections occur.

Use the following as guiding criteria (in this order):
1. Collateral Connections
2. Tortuosity
3. Size
4. Angle of connection (CTSA)

Select frames to clarify connection.

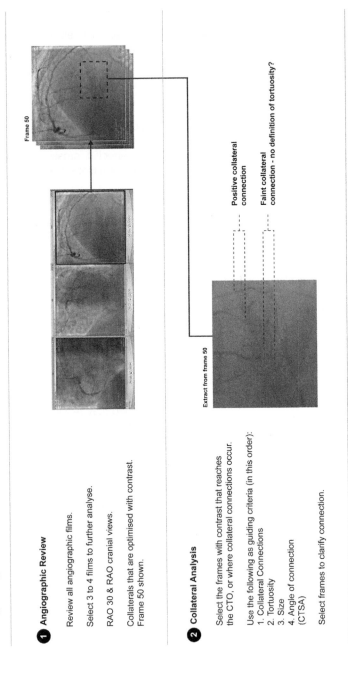

Frame 50

Extract from frame 50

Positive collateral connection

Faint collateral connection - no definition of tortuosity?

Fig. 6. An image algorithm which we have used to facilitate septal crossing.

3 Collateral Enhancement

Alter image contrast / brightness to provide more collateral detail.

In some cases inverting the image (negative) can provide more information whilst increasing contrast and / or brightness.

Alternatively, using image enhancing software can give even further detail and definition.

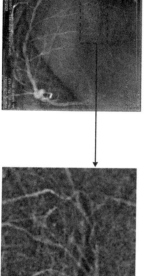

Frame 50 Inverted (negative)

Positive collateral connection with increased definition of septal tortuosity

4 Collateral Road Map

Before selecting the enhanced image as THE road map - check angulation of connecting collaterals.

In some cases a combination of films will be required to confirm CTSA.

Play the films next to the enhanced still image created in stage 1 using two monitors.

Identify the collaterals in terms of priority 1.

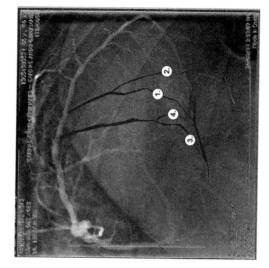

Fig. 6. (*continued*)

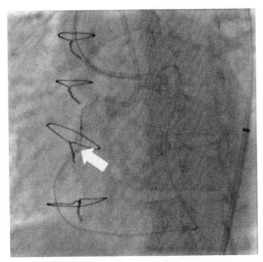

Retrograde knuckle wire with Corsair support

Fig. 7. The use of a "knuckle" wire helps to clarify anatomic ambiguity and reduces the risk of wire exit.

Crossability

Although there is a relationship between operator experience and septal crossability, there still remains a significant degree of unpredictability. The larger studies report a failure-to-cross rate of about 25%[3] in experienced retrograde operators in selected cases, suggesting that this aspect of the procedure remains a significant potential limiter of success. Some attempts have been made to determine reasons for failure to cross, and these are outlined here.

Tortuosity

Tortuosity is probably the most reliable predictor of failure to cross, but is difficult to assess. A related characteristic is distensibility, which can be assessed by the way the septal channel either remains coiled throughout the cardiac cycle or uncoils during diastole. Distensibility may be used as a surrogate marker for crossability, which uncoil during diastole cc then being more crossable.

Size

Size is not a reliable way to assess crossability, although there may be some relationship between tortuosity and size, with larger septal channels tending to be more tortuous. Indeed it is possible to cross very small or even invisible cc, a precept that underlines the principle of "septal surfing," described later.

Angle of entry

Angle of entry may be an important limiter, with very sharply angulated septal channels being difficult to access, for both wires and subsequent microcatheters. The angle of the distal donor vessel should also be considered; if this is very acute, passage of the microcatheter can sometimes result in kinking of the distal donor vessel and, in turn, ischemia. If this is considered to be a possibility, placing a wire in the distal donor vessel is advisable. The angle at the base of the heart (for LAD to RCA connections), if acute, can also be a significant limiter for both wire and microcatheter passage.

Technique for Septal Collateral Wiring

As the retrograde technique has evolved, it has changed from dilatation of the septal collaterals with balloons to the primary use of the corsair catheter, also called a channel dilator. It has several characteristics, which enable it to be a very effective retrograde tool (**Fig. 9**), and is used as the microcatheter of choice in most retrograde procedures. A workhorse wire is used to access the cc of choice and the corsair advanced with a rotational movement (it can be turned both counterclockwise and clockwise, up to a maximum of 10 turns in each direction before the torque is released). The wire is then carefully removed while simultaneously injecting saline (to prevent air embolus). A soft wire with a very small distal curve is used to cannulate the septal channels (current preferred wires are Sion, Fielder FC [Asahi Intecc], Whisper [Abbot Vascular] or, if very small channels, Fielder XT [Asahi Intecc]). The precept underlying septal surfing is the use of

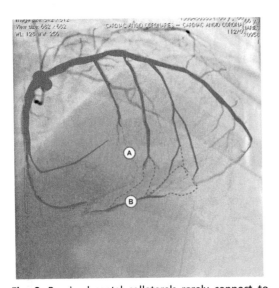

Fig. 8. Proximal septal collaterals rarely connect to the PDA branch of the RCA, but can connect (as in this case) to the PLV (collateral A). Collateral connections are demonstrated to the PDA (collateral pathway B).

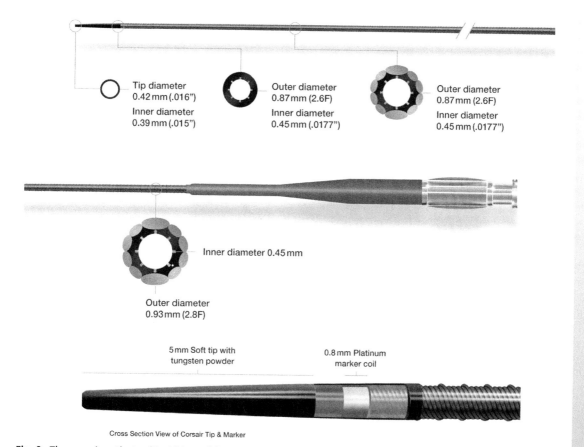

Tip diameter
0.42 mm (.016")
Inner diameter
0.39 mm (.015")

Outer diameter
0.87 mm (2.6F)
Inner diameter
0.45 mm (.0177")

Outer diameter
0.87 mm (2.6F)
Inner diameter
0.45 mm (.0177")

Inner diameter 0.45 mm

Outer diameter
0.93 mm (2.8F)

5 mm Soft tip with
tungsten powder

0.8 mm Platinum
marker coil

Cross Section View of Corsair Tip & Marker

Fig. 9. The corsair catheter (Asahi Intecc) has several features which contribute to its use as the retrograde catheter of choice.

the relatively random, or at least poorly defined, septal connections. Rarely septal connections are visible and contiguous, in which case wiring of these channels is more directed. Septal surfing involves advancing the wire of choice relatively quickly until resistance is felt or the wire advances into the distal CTO. In the event of resistance being felt, the wire is quickly redirected to find an alternative channel. If after several passes the distal CTO has not been achieved, the septal connection should be visualized by contrast (via 2-mL Luer-lock syringe). If this confirms a good connection to the distal vessel, the wire should be reshaped and further attempts made; if not, an alternative septal connection should be sought (**Fig. 10**). Proximal septal access is best achieved in a cranial projection (often RAO cranial), whereas access to the distal CTO is best appreciated in RAO 30° or RAO caudal. Confirmation of the wire crossing to the RCA can be checked in left anterior oblique (LAO) 30° or LAO cranial, and is associated with a change in the distal wire movement from the relatively fixed movement of the distal wire tip seen within the septum to a to-and-fro movement mediated by cardiac movement.

It is not uncommon in the process of septal wiring for the wire to enter the right ventricle (from very proximal septal perforators), left ventricle, or even the venous system. This scenario may be recognized (in the first 2 cases) by sudden rapid and large deviations in wire-tip movement. These deviations, as long as recognized and not followed by microcatheters/balloons, are entirely benign and are a consequence of existing intracardiac connections.

Technique for Crossing Septal cc Following Wire Crossing

Once the wire has accessed the distal CTO, it should be advanced rapidly to the level of the distal cap to facilitate subsequent advancement of the microcatheter/balloon. To cross the cc the corsair catheter should be torqued clockwise and anticlockwise (a maximum of 10 rotations in each direction) while applying a small amount of forward push. At the same time a minor amount of traction should be applied on the wire. This process may be rather slow and is often facilitated by cardiac motion. In approximately 10% of cases the corsair may fail to cross: in this situation the

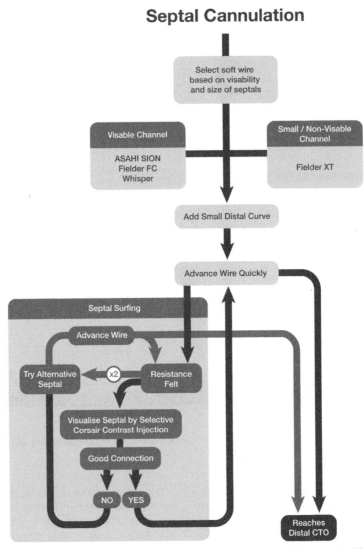

Fig. 10. An algorithm for septal "surfing" is demonstrated: this techniques relies on a suitable wire being rapidly directed (and redirected) towards the CTO vessel until resistance is felt.

options include up-titrating support, by using balloon-anchor techniques or a Guideliner catheter (Vascular Solutions Inc, Minneapolis, MN, USA), or by using a long, small balloon to dilate the cc. Occasionally, if the case is prolonged or the corsair catheter excessively torqued, it can become more adherent to the wire and less effective, requiring it to be replaced.

EPICARDIAL COLLATERALS

The principles of crossing epicardial collaterals are different. There is no role for septal surfing; instead the wire is carefully manipulated to follow what are often very tortuous channels. It is very important in

such situations to carefully assess the safety of cc crossing, given that perforation in the context of an intact pericardium may result in pericardial tamponade. In general, larger epicardial channels are safer and more likely to permit the passage of equipment. The authors believe it is mandatory to take careful selective injections via the microcatheter of choice, in at least 2 orthogonal views, which then can be used as "road maps" to assess wire progress.

Technique for Epicardial Collateral Wiring

A soft wire, currently the wire of choice in Europe and Japan, is the Sion wire (Asahi Intecc). As this is not available in the United States, alternatives include the Fielder FC (Asahi Intecc) or Whisper wire (Abbott Vascular). With an angulation at the very distal tip of approximately 30° the wire is advanced into the cc beyond the first couple of curves and is then followed by the corsair catheter, ensuring that it does not get too close to the tip or "overtake" the wire. The corsair catheter is advanced by rotating in both directions and will "straighten" the cc in sections, thus permitting steady advancement of the wire. Movement of the wire can often be very sudden and rapid and is facilitated by cardiac movement, which can in turn reduce wire control. It is important to confirm wire position before corsair advancement. Correct positioning can be achieved by reference to the road maps already created or by direct injection through the microcatheter. Once the wire has reached the distal vessel, it should be advanced to the distal cap of the CTO to further facilitate delivery of the microcatheter.

Advancing to the Proximal Cap and Setting Up a Base of Operations

The objective after crossing the cc is to arrive, as quickly and safely as possible, at the proximal cap of the CTO, referred to as the base of operations (**Fig. 11**). Although this can occasionally be achieved by simple wiring with the relatively soft wire used for cc crossing, it is much more common to encounter significant resistance at the distal cap of the CTO. This being the case, the microcatheter should be advanced as far as possible to maximize backup support. The wire chosen next will depend on the length of the CTO and morphology of the

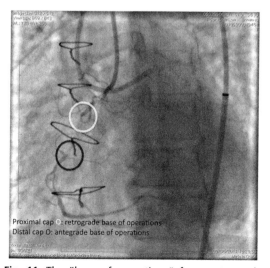

Fig. 11. The "base of operations" for a retrograde procedure is the proximal cap of the CTO.

distal cap. If the CTO is relatively short (<20 mm) and/or there is a side branch at the distal cap, a stiff penetrative wire should be chosen (Confienza 12 g Pro [Ashai Intecc], Progress 200 T [Abbott Vascular], Provia 15 g [Medtronic, Minneapolis, MN, USA]). The objective should either be direct wiring (in the case of a short CTO without significant anatomic ambiguity) or penetration far enough into the CTO to permit delivery of the microcatheter. This being achieved, a polymer-coated wire (Pilot 200) should be chosen and the wire "knuckled" (as previously described), then advanced to the level of the proximal cap with the microcatheter being advanced as close to the knuckle as possible. The knuckle can be used as a primary strategy if there is not a side branch at the distal cap, but still often requires the use of a penetrative wire to create vessel injury first. A knuckled wire is of particular help in a long CTO or one with significant anatomic ambiguity, where it can transverse long segments of occlusions rapidly with a low risk of vessel perforation.

Crossing the CTO

Direct wiring is said to be possible in approximately 25% of cases, but it is the view of the authors that with appropriate wire escalation this figure is nearer to 50%. The key to successful, safe wiring is to minimize anatomic ambiguity, which is best achieved by placing the microcatheter as close to the proximal cap as possible (usually by the use of a knuckle wire, as described earlier) and then replacing the knuckle wire with a penetrative wire (also described above). This wire should have an angulation of approximately 45° placed about 8 mm from the tip (ie, a longer curve and more angulation than a CTO curve), which should be directed toward the proximal vessel guided by gentle antegrade injections.

SUMMARY

Retrograde access has resulted in improved procedural success in the treatment of CTOs, but requires a thorough understanding of the principles involved and careful planning. The adage "failure to plan equals planning to fail" is highly applicable here. The challenges encountered in treating these highly resistant lesions require a familiarity with a range of supportive techniques and an ability to be flexible in both strategy and approach. It is the authors' view that this is best achieved by a combination of a sound basis of theoretical knowledge combined with the use of dedicated courses and experienced proctors.

ACKNOWLEDGMENTS

The authors give special thanks to Adrian Brown from Vascular Perspectives for his invaluable help with image support and his new perspective on these challenging issues.

SUPPLEMENTARY DATA

Supplementary data related to this article can be found online at doi:10.1016/j.iccl.2012.05.001.

REFERENCES

1. Serruys PW, Morice MC, Kappetein AP, et al. Percutaneous coronary intervention versus coronary-artery bypass grafting for severe coronary artery disease. N Engl J Med 2009;360:961–72.

2. Kahn JK, Hartzler GO. Retrograde coronary angioplasty of isolated arterial segments through saphenous vein bypass grafts. Cathet Cardiovasc Diagn 1990;20:88–93.

3. Rathore S, Katoh O, Matsuo H, et al. Retrograde percutaneous recanalization of chronic total occlusion of the coronary arteries: procedural outcomes and predictors of success in contemporary practice. Circ Cardiovasc Interv 2009;2:124–32.

4. Galassi AR, Tomasello SD, Reifart N, et al. In-hospital outcomes of percutaneous coronary intervention in patients with chronic total occlusion: insights from the ERCTO (European Registry of Chronic Total Occlusion) registry. EuroIntervention 2011;7(4):472–9.

5. Tsujita K, Maehara A, Mintz GS, et al. Intravascular ultrasound comparison of the retrograde versus antegrade approach to percutaneous intervention for chronic total coronary occlusions. JACC Cardiovasc Interv 2009;2:846–54.

6. Katsuragawa M, Fujiwara H, Miyamae M, et al. Histologic studies in percutaneous transluminal coronary angioplasty for chronic total occlusion: comparison of tapering and abrupt types of occlusion and short and long occluded segments. J Am Coll Cardiol 1993;21:604–11.

7. Widimsky P, Straka Z, Stros P, et al. One-year coronary bypass graft patency: a randomized comparison between off-pump and on-pump surgery angiographic results of the PRAGUE-4 trial. Circulation 2004;110(22):3418–23.

8. Werner GS, Ferrari M, Heinke S, et al. Angiographic assessment of collateral connections in comparison with invasively determined collateral function in chronic coronary occlusions. Circulation 2003;107:1972–7.

Retrograde Dissection Reentry for Coronary Chronic Total Occlusions

Tony J. DeMartini, MD

KEYWORDS

- Chronic total occlusion • Percutaneous coronary intervention • Retrograde technique
- Reverse CART

KEY POINTS

- The retrograde technique is an important tool for overall successful percutaneous coronary intervention (PCI) of chronic total occlusions (CTOs).
- Reverse controlled antegrade and retrograde subintimal tracking (rCART) is the most frequently used retrograde technique.
- Compliance with the basic steps of rCART provides an efficient and a safe approach for successful retrograde coronary PCI of CTO.

INTRODUCTION

The retrograde technique is an important skill set for improving the overall success of percutaneous coronary intervention of chronic total occlusions (CTOs). A subset of CTOs that cannot be performed with an antegrade-only approach exists. An antegrade-only approach results in success rates of 60% to 70%.[1] The retrograde approach was first introduced by Japanese operators[2,3] and was more widely adopted with the introduction of the Corsair catheter (Asahi Intecc, Nagoya, Japan).[4]

The retrograde dissection reentry is an approach that has evolved with advances in technology and improvements in technique. The approach involves both antegrade access to the proximal cap and retrograde access to the distal cap of a CTO.[5] The reverse controlled antegrade and retrograde subintimal tracking (rCART) is the most common technique used in North America.

The technique uses the subintimal/subadventitial space to connect the proximal true lumen to the distal true lumen. Multiple variations of the rCART have been developed, but the principles of the procedure remain the same.

TECHNIQUE

The rCART is a specific sequence of steps that uses the subintimal space to provide an efficient technique to connect the proximal true lumen to the distal true lumen. This technique requires retrograde access to the distal cap of the CTO, which is discussed elsewhere in this issue. Retrograde access is in the distal true lumen to the point of the distal cap. A diagram of basic CTO anatomy is provided in **Fig. 1** for reference of anatomic descriptions.

The guidewire set for CTO has been honed to 4 wires: the Fielder XT (Asahi Intecc, Nagoya, Japan), the Fielder FC (Asahi Intecc, Nagoya, Japan), the Pilot 200 (Abbott Vascular, Santa Clara, CA, USA), and the Confianza Pro 12 (Asahi Intecc, Nagoya, Japan), and each guidewire has a specific purpose in performing the rCART procedure.

Disclosures: Speakers Bureau: Vascular Solutions, Boston Scientific; Speakers Bureau and Proctor: Bridgepoint Medical, Abbott Vascular.
Prairie Cardiovascular Consultants, 401 East Carpenter, Springfield, IL 62702, USA
E-mail address: ctoskrat@comcast.net

Intervent Cardiol Clin 1 (2012) 339–344
doi:10.1016/j.iccl.2012.04.008
2211-7458/12/$ – see front matter © 2012 Elsevier Inc. All rights reserved.

interventional.theclinics.com

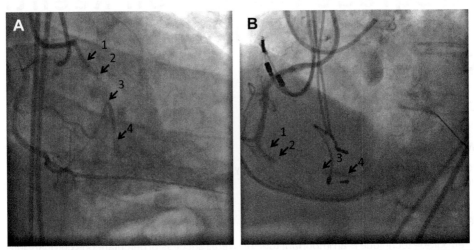

Fig. 1. Basic anatomy of a CTO. (*A*) Circumflex with right coronary artery collaterals. (*B*) Occluded RCA with left to right and right to right collaterals. 1, proximal true lumen; 2, proximal cap; 3, distal cap; 4, distal true lumen.

The Fielder XT is used to probe for microchannels and knuckle both the antegrade and retrograde. The Fielder FC is used to gain retrograde access via collaterals and, occasionally, for wiring the true lumen after performing rCART. The Pilot 200 is used for knuckling and wiring the true lumen. The Confianza Pro 12 is used for crossing resistant areas when the course of the vessel is known and for reentering the true lumen from the subintimal space.

The rCART steps include retrograde dissection in the subintimal space past the distal cap, advancement of a retrograde support catheter over the dissection wire to near the proximal cap, antegrade subintimal access to a point distal to the retrograde support catheter, and deployment of an antegrade balloon in the subintimal space next to the retrograde support catheter with subsequent connection of the subintimal space and the retrograde wiring from the support catheter into the proximal true lumen.

Step 1. Retrograde Dissection

A retrograde dissection plan can be initiated by several approaches (**Fig. 2**). A soft tapered polymer jacketed wire (Fielder XT) can be used to probe for a microchannel, or a knuckle wire may allow access to the subintimal space. If the Fielder XT is unsuccessful, a polymer jacketed nontapered wire (Pilot 200) would be used next in an attempt to allow the knuckle wire to access the

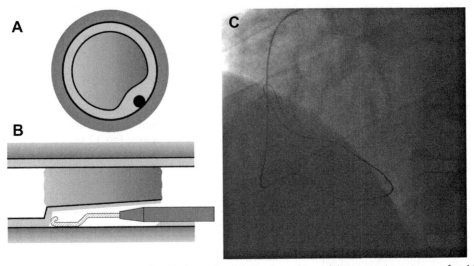

Fig. 2. (*A*) Cross-sectional cartoon of initiation of subintimal tracking. (*B*) Long-axis cartoon of subintimal tracking. (*C*) Retrograde knuckle wire advanced to the proximal cap of coronary CTO.

subintimal space. In the event that the knuckle wire cannot penetrate the subintimal space, a stiff tapered wire (Confianza Pro 12) may be needed. Caution should be exercised, and the wire should only be advanced by a short distance (5–10 mm). After the distal cap is crossed with a wire, the support catheter (preferably the Corsair catheter) should be advanced past the distal cap.

The knuckle wire technique is used to dissect the artery from the distal cap to the proximal cap. A knuckle wire is a prolapsed wire that is advanced without torquing. The soft leading edge of the wire is unlikely to perforate the vessel because it takes the path of least resistance, which is the subintimal plane. Either a jacketed tapered or a jacketed nontapered wire can be used. The knuckle wire usually starts dissecting at the transition point from the soft tip to the stiffer shaft. As the wire is advanced, the support catheter should be kept within 10 to 20 mm of the tip of the knuckle to provide support.

A common pitfall is the attempt to wire the lesion in a "true lumen to true lumen" manner. Although this may be feasible, it most commonly leads to prolonged case times as well as increased contrast and radiation usage.

Step 2. Antegrade Dissection

A common reason for the retrograde approach is an ambiguous proximal cap. Once the retrograde dissection is complete, the proximal cap is more obvious. At present, an antegrade dissection technique is used; similar to the retrograde technique, a wire escalation approach is used. In addition to removing the ambiguity of the proximal cap, the retrograde wire also provides an outline of the course of the vessel.

The rCART technique may also be used if the antegrade dissection reentry attempt has been unsuccessful.

The antegrade wire is advanced into the CTO, and the balloon catheter is then advanced in the antegrade direction. The antegrade balloon should be 15 to 20 mm in length and sized to match the normal vessel lumen. A smaller balloon or Tornus catheter (Asahi Intecc, Nagoya, Japan) may be initially required to modify the proximal cap to deliver balloons with a higher crossing profile.

Intravascular ultrasonography may be used to size the vessel and balloon if proximal disease makes sizing difficult.

Once antegrade dissection has been performed, injections through the antegrade guide catheter should be avoided, because this can cause a hydraulic dissection and a compromise of the distal vascular bed.

Step 3. Creating a Common Subintimal Space

The antegrade balloon is positioned such that the tip of the retrograde support catheter is in the midportion of the antegrade balloon (**Figs. 3–5**). The balloon is then deployed to give a diameter equal to the size of the vessel. The most common reason for failure is an undersized balloon. The key concept is the creation of a common subintimal space. Before balloon inflation, the balloon and the retrograde support catheter may appear up to 4 to 5 mm apart on fluoroscopy, yet they are both in the subintimal space. The important aspect is not the distance between the 2 devices but that

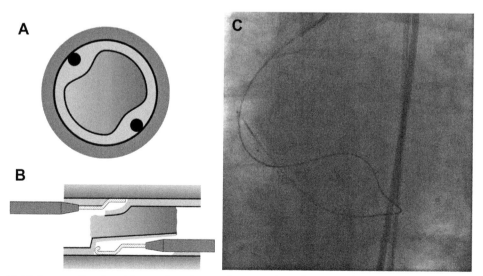

Fig. 3. (*A, B*) Cross-sectional and long-axis cartoons of antegrade and retrograde wires and devices in the subintimal space. (*C*) Retrograde support catheter near proximal cap with antegrade knuckle wire and balloon next to the support catheter.

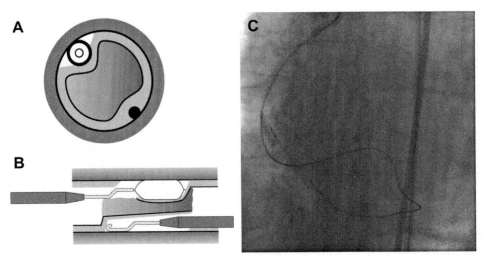

Fig. 4. (*A, B*) Cross-sectional and long-axis cartoons of antegrade balloon that are either undersized or underdeployed, with persistent tissue between the 2 subintimal locations. (*C*) Inflated balloon next to the retrograde support catheter, with tissue plane remaining between the 2 devices.

both are within the vessel architecture. With balloon inflation, the true lumen is moved aside to the point where the 2 subintimal spaces become 1 space. The common space is not created if an undersized balloon is used.

When the balloon is inflated, there should be no space between the balloon and the support catheter. If a gap exists (see **Fig. 4**), then there remains tissue between the 2 and the common space does not exist. In this instance, either a higher inflation pressure is required or a larger diameter balloon needs to be used.

After successful elimination of any gap between the devices, a common space is created (see **Fig. 5**). On deflation of the balloon, the support catheter can be seen "dropping" into the potential space created by the balloon (**Fig. 6**). When this occurs, there exists a continuous pathway from the distal true lumen, through the subintimal space, and into the proximal true lumen. A jacketed nontapered wire is then used to traverse the remaining subintimal space created by the balloon into the true lumen. Subsequently, the retrograde wire in the proximal true lumen can be either used to wire the antegrade guide catheter or is snared via the antegrade guide catheter. After externalization, the procedure can be completed using conventional angioplasty techniques.

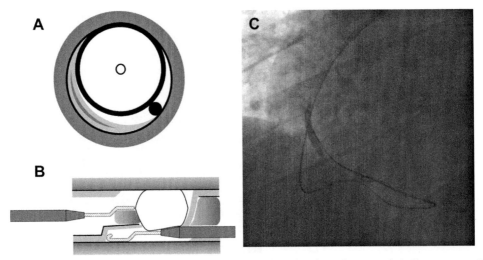

Fig. 5. (*A, B*) Cross-sectional and long-axis views of properly inflated and sized antegrade balloon connecting the 2 subintimal spaces. (*C*) Retrograde support catheter next to the antegrade balloon, with no residual space between the devices.

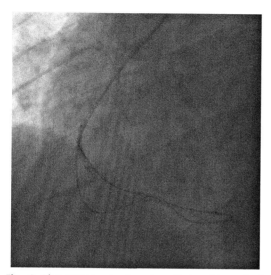

Fig. 6. The retrograde Corsair catheter "dropping" into the space left by the antegrade balloon, forming a common subintimal space.

MODES OF FAILURE

The benefits of the rCART technique are that it is predictable and reproducible. Failure occurs when there are deviations from the outlined approach. Prolonged attempts to wire the proximal true lumen commonly lead to extended contrast and radiation exposure. This causes the case to stall and leads to extended laboratory time.

Undersizing the antegrade balloon makes the creation of a common subintimal space much more difficult. Choosing appropriately sized balloons allows for an efficient and a safe procedure.

Reentry is very difficult when the retrograde wire and support catheter are in the subintimal space and the antegrade balloon is in the true lumen. Unlike the antegrade dissection reentry technique, there is no device that is dedicated to this approach. Despite appropriately sized balloons, a common space is not created and reentry with the retrograde wire crossing tissue must occur to enter into the true lumen. This approach is an option if antegrade subintimal access is not possible but is suboptimal with respect to efficiency.

VARIATIONS IN TECHNIQUE

Variations in the technique involve differences in the antegrade approach. The subintimal space can either compress or collapse after antegrade balloon inflation and deflation. This makes wiring the true lumen, even with a continuous subintimal connection, more difficult. There are 2 main solutions to avoid this compression.

After antegrade balloon inflation, a stent may be deployed from the antegrade true lumen into the antegrade subintimal space. This provides scaffolding and may facilitate retrograde wiring. This technique is referred to as stent rCART. Caution should be exercised because this is a definitive step. Even if the procedure is ultimately unsuccessful, a permanent connection has been made from the antegrade true lumen to the subintimal space. Repeated attempts are hampered with this technique.

An alternative method is to use a GuideLiner mother and child catheter (Vascular Solutions, Minneapolis, MN, USA) to scaffold open the subintimal space. The GuideLiner has several advantages over the stent rCART. After the GuideLiner is placed into the subintimal space, it provides a continuous conduit to the antegrade guide. This removes issues of creating a new dissection plane or wiring into side branches. Unlike a stent, a catheter may be removed or repositioned if the connection between the antegrade and the retrograde true lumens is unsuccessful.

Intravascular ultrasonography may be required if either the antegrade or retrograde wire is in the true lumen. This is rarely necessary if both systems exist in the subintimal space.

The controlled antegrade and retrograde subintimal tracking technique may also be used. This technique is similar to rCART except that the balloon inflation is done from the retrograde system, and wiring from the proximal true lumen to the distal true lumen occurs in an antegrade direction. The use of the Corsair catheter has greatly decreased the need for this technique.

SUMMARY

The retrograde technique is an important tool for the overall success of CTO angioplasty. The rCART technique is the most frequently used approach for retrograde dissection reentry and can be used as a primary approach or as an alternative after an unsuccessful primary antegrade dissection reentry approach.

Variations of this technique, mostly with regard to the antegrade aspect, exist as alternatives for success in approaches in which the basic technique is failing. Compliance with the basic outlined steps allows for efficient, reproducible, and successful outcomes.

REFERENCES

1. Joyal D, Afilalo J, Rinfret S. Effectiveness of recanalization of chronic total occlusions: a systematic review and meta-analysis. Am Heart J 2010;160:179–87.

2. Surmely JF, Tsuchikane E, Katoh O, et al. New concept for CTO recanalization using controlled antegrade and retrograde subintimal tracking: the CART technique. J Invasive Cardiol 2006;18:334–8.

3. Surmely JF, Katoh O, Tsuchikane E, et al. Coronary septal collaterals as an access for retrograde approach in the percutaneous treatment of coronary chronic total occlusions. Catheter Cardiovasc Interv 2007;69:826–32.

4. Tsuchikane E, Katoh O, Kimura M, et al. The first clinical experience with a novel catheter for collateral channel tracking in retrograde approach for chronic coronary total occlusions. JACC Cardiovasc Interv 2010;3:165–71.

5. Joyal D, Thompson CA, Grantham JA, et al. The retrograde technique for recanalization of chronic total occlusions: a step-by-step approach. JACC Cardiovasc Interv 2012;5:1–11.

The Final Steps of the Retrograde Technique
Wire Externalization, Stenting, and Wire Removal

J. Aaron Grantham, MD

KEYWORDS

- Retrograde • Stenting • Externalization • Guidewire

KEY POINTS

- Place the retrograde crossing wire and collateral microcatheter into the antegrade guide.
- Exchange the crossing wire for the externalization wire.
- Externalize the wire and hook up the antegrade flush system.
- The final treatment of the lesion is with standard ballooning and stenting.
- Remove the externalized guidewire and collateral microcatheter.

A guidewire can be externalized after retrograde lesion crossing. An externalized guidewire provides excellent support for ballooning and stenting. There are 5 key steps in wire externalization:

1. Placing the retrograde crossing wire and collateral microcatheter into the antegrade guide
2. Exchanging the crossing wire for the externalization wire
3. Externalizing the wire and hooking up the antegrade flush system
4. Final treatment of the lesion with standard ballooning and stenting
5. Removal of the externalized guidewire and collateral microcatheter.

PLACING THE CROSSING WIRE AND COLLATERAL MICROCATHETER IN THE ANTEGRADE GUIDE

After crossing the chronic total occlusion (CTO) lesion with a crossing wire or using controlled antegrade and retrograde tracking (CART) or reverse CART dissection and reentry techniques, establish coaxial antegrade guide positioning. An attempt can then be made to advance the retrograde crossing wire into the antegrade guide. It does not matter which wire is used to cross the lesion: a short or long wire, a jacketed or nonjacketed wire, or a tapered or nontapered wire. The only caution is that when stiff and tapered wires are used, if there is a long distance between the antegrade cap and the antegrade guide, the microcatheter (usually the Corsair channel dilator; Asahi Intecc, Nagoya, Japan) should be advanced across the lesion and the tapered and stiff wires should be exchanged for workhorse-type wires to avoid dissection or perforation of a relatively nondiseased segment of the vessel.

The microcatheter should be placed soon after the wire has been placed within the antegrade guide. The channel dilator should be positioned 5 to 7 cm within the guide. The delivery of the channel dilator can be facilitated by trapping the retrograde wire inside the antegrade guide using a balloon. Careful attention has to be paid to the retrograde guide when it is trapped inside the antegrade guide. With traction on the crossing wire,

University of Missouri Kansas City, Saint Luke's Mid America Heart Institute, 4401 Wornall Road, MAHI 5th Floor, Kansas City, MO 64111, USA
E-mail address: jgrantham@saint-lukes.org

Intervent Cardiol Clin 1 (2012) 345–348
doi:10.1016/j.iccl.2012.04.007
2211-7458/12/$ – see front matter © 2012 Elsevier Inc. All rights reserved.

especially when it is trapped inside the antegrade guide, the retrograde guide will be pulled into the donor vessel potentially dissecting or occluding that vessel. In addition, tension will develop in the collateral system, which can result in collateral shearing; rupture; or, even worse, slicing of the heart. The retrograde wire should almost never be pulled, only pushed, to avoid this potentially catastrophic complication.

EXCHANGING THE CROSSING WIRE FOR THE EXTERNALIZATION WIRE

The crossing wire can be removed and exchanged for an externalization wire after the microcatheter is delivered into the antegrade guide. There are 3 examples of good externalization wires: the first is a 335-cm 0.014" peripheral rotational atherectomy wire called the ViperWire Advance (Cardiovascular Systems Inc, St Paul, MN, USA), the second is a 330-cm 0.010" coronary rotational atherectomy wire called the RotaWire (Boston Scientific, Natick, MA, USA), and the third is a 330-cm 0.010" purpose-built retrograde wire called the RG3 (Asahi Intecc, Nagoya, Japan). These 3 wires each have limitations. The ViperWire is 0.014 in, extraordinarily stiff, and is often difficult to pass through very tortuous collaterals. This has largely been overcome by flushing the channel dilator with Rotaglide solution (Boston Scientific, Natick, MA, USA) before insertion of the externalization wire. The RotaWire is too flimsy, too prone to kinking, and not very useful for externalization but can be used as a last resort if no other wires are available in long lengths. The RG3 is the optimal wire. The only limitation is that the shaft is not as stiff as a standard coronary wire and therefore it is less able to support balloons and stents after externalization; the RG3 is not available in the United States.

Despite coaxial rotation of the antegrade guide, passing the retrograde wire into the guide sometimes fails. This is not uncommon in aorto-ostial lesions or extremely tortuous vessels, or whenever there is poor retrograde guidewire control or the vessel caliber is much larger than the antegrade guide. Difficulty in wiring the antegrade guide can be overcome by snaring.

After 4 to 5 passes with the retrograde wire and perhaps a reshaping or two, snaring should be done quickly after wiring the guide. Externalization should not take more than 5 minutes, and wiring the guide should not consume more than 2 to 3 minutes of the procedure time. The 3-snare system, commonly referred to as a tulip snare (EN Snare; Merit Medical Systems, South Jordan, UT, USA), is the most useful snaring system for externalization of a long guidewire during a retrograde procedure. The larger the snare the better. An 18 × 30 mm EN Snare snare, which is 6 French compatible, is preferred.

The EN Snare 3-snare system comes with a delivery catheter, but it is not necessary to use it in retrograde externalization. The key components are the snare wire, the introducer, and the torquing device (**Fig. 1**). Simply pull the snare back into the introducer, and insert the introducer into the antegrade copilot. Advance the snare out the end of the antegrade guide and position it as near to the coronary ostium as possible. After positioning the snare at the ostium of the antegrade coronary artery (**Fig. 2**), advance the retrograde wire out of the coronary ostium and pull back on the snare. The snare catches the wire, sweeping it into the antegrade guide and repositioning the antegrade guide back to the ostium of the occluded vessel.

During snaring, the tips and tricks shown in **Box 1** should be kept in mind.

Ipsilateral collateral use of the retrograde procedure poses a unique challenge to wire externalization. Wire externalization can be done as long as an 8 French guiding system is used (**Fig. 3**). When efficient guide wiring is not possible, snaring is not an option. When the wire can be advanced into the guiding catheter, advance the Corsair back into the single guide. The channel-crossing catheter has effectively gone retrograde through the collateral and back into the antegrade guide. Remove the crossing wire, flush the Corsair with Rotaglide solution, and then push the externalization wire out of the guiding catheter hub. Reconnect with the steps described subsequently. Back the Corsair out to allow antegrade rapid exchange treatment. Again, when efficient wiring is not possible, snaring is not an option. The solution to this challenge is to place a second or a ping-pong guiding system.

EXTERNALIZING THE WIRE AND HOOKING UP THE ANTEGRADE COPILOT SYSTEM

As the externalized wire approaches the antegrade guiding hub, detach the copilot, place a finger over the hub of the antegrade guide, and

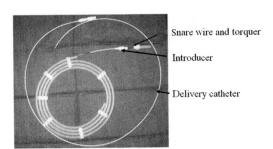

Snare wire and torquer

Introducer

Delivery catheter

Fig. 1. The EN Snare 3-snare system.

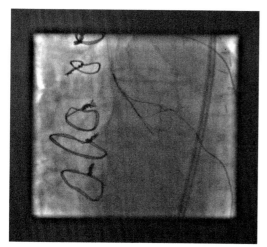

Fig. 2. Alignment of the snare via the antegrade guide with the left main coronary artery. The Corsair has passed from a degenerated graft retrograde through the left circumflex, then out of the left main coronary artery. The crossing wire extends into the aorta and through the snare.

flushing. Flushing after reverse CART can result in hydraulic propagation of the intentional dissection. Continue externalizing 20 to 30 cm of the wire. When snaring has been performed, push the wire through the antegrade copilot. Cut the bent end of the snared wire, back up the channel dilator to allow antegrade lesion treatment but always protect the collateral; never pull the Corsair or the crossing catheter all the way out of the recipient vessel.

FINAL TREATMENT

After the wire has been externalized 20 to 30 cm, there is more than enough to perform balloon and stent treatment with rapid exchange gear via the antegrade guide. Back up the channel dilator to allow sufficient room to deliver gear antegrade. Use retrograde injections to visualize the distal landing zone for stents. The following precautions must be kept in mind:

1. Never leave an externalized wire unprotected by a catheter in a tortuous collateral. Always leave the channel dilator or channel-crossing catheter over the stiff wire, which is still within the collateral.
2. Never pull either end of the externalized wire unless the collateral that it has crossed is protected with a catheter, and only do this when

wait for the retrograde wire to tap it. Once the tap of the retrograde wire is felt, push the retrograde wire 5 to 7 cm out of the guide. Place a wire introducer into the antegrade copilot and thread the externalized soft tip of the wire through the introducer (**Fig. 4**). Then, slide the introducer and copilot over the wire and reconnect it without

---

Box 1
Tips and tricks for snaring

1. Always snare the wire that is to be externalized. Pulling the externalized wire into the guide sometimes bends the wire to a significant degree. Retraction or removal of these severely bent wires can be very difficult. Therefore, once the clinician has committed to snaring a wire, it should be a wire that is of sufficient length to be pulled all the way through and externalized (>300 cm). This means that the Corsair should be delivered into the aorta; then the crossing wire should be removed and the Corsair flushed, followed by advancement of the externalization wire. The externalization wire is snared, if needed, and then passed all the way through the antegrade guide.

2. Always snare the soft part of the wire. This is necessary because snaring on the stiff portion of most externalization wires results in kinking, which can result in shearing of the antegrade guide tip. In addition, once the extra support wire is taken and pulled into the antegrade guide, removing it from the Corsair is impossible. Caution should be exercised when snaring the soft portion of the wire. These wires are generally coiled and can unravel. The key is to try to sweep the wire gently into the guide under continuous fluoroscopic observation. A pop or release of the wire may represent uncoiling.

3. Once snared, the externalization wire can be rapidly advanced through the system all the way out of the copilot. Most of the pressure within the system should come from pushing. Gentle continuous traction can be placed on the snare to facilitate movement of the wire through the system and out of the antegrade guiding catheter, but care must be taken to avoid cinching the guides deep into the coronary arteries. Gently push the wire completely through the copilot, remove from the snare, and cut off the bent end of the wire to facilitate the loading of rapid exchange balloons and stents.

4. Gently sweep the wire into the antegrade catheter and take care not to unravel the coils. If a polymer-jacketed wire has been snared, the polymer jacket can be stripped. Therefore after externalization, back bleeding is of paramount importance.

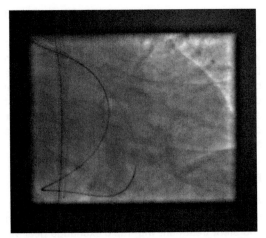

Fig. 3. Ipsilateral wiring of the guide. When wiring fails, a second ping-pong guide can be placed to allow snaring.

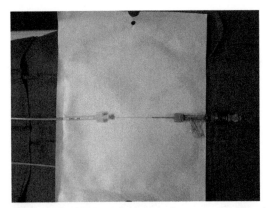

Fig. 4. Configuration of the gear for reattachment of the flush system to the antegrade guide.

both guides are visible. Pushing is always permitted but it still needs to be done with protection of the collaterals.
3. Never allow antegrade balloons or catheters to meet retrograde balloons or catheters on the same externalized guidewire. In the past, this has resulted in locking of the 2 catheters, making extraction of the catheters impossible except by surgical extraction.

REMOVAL OF THE EXTERNALIZED GUIDEWIRE AND CORSAIR CHANNEL DILATOR

After stenting, removal of the device is the final step in wire externalization. To remove the wire, the channel dilator should be readvanced to the antegrade guide. Both guiding catheters should then be disengaged from the coronary ostium and pulled back 3 to 4 cm into the aorta because, when the externalized wire is retracted, the guides tend to be pulled into the coronary ostium. This problem can be prevented if the technique is begun with retracted guides and the guides are held at the sheath hub. To disengage the retrograde guiding catheter, push the channel dilator and slide the guide out. To disengage the antegrade guiding catheter, simply push the externalized portion of the wire coming out of the antegrade guide. Once guiding catheter control

has been established, pull the externalized wire back from where it came. It is important that the wire is not kinked to facilitate retraction. Once the externalized wire has been completely removed, remove the channel dilator with clockwise rotation. It is not necessary to leave the wire within the channel dilator to retract it but some advocate leaving some part of the wire so that the collateral can be accessed easily in the event of a collateral channel rupture. This access could help to more rapidly coil the wire or otherwise manage this complication.

SUMMARY

Wire externalization provides excellent support for the treatment of CTO lesions that are long calcified, tortuous, and difficult to treat. There are 5 key steps to wire externalization:

1. Wiring the antegrade guide and following it with the channel dilator; this may require snaring
2. Exchanging the crossing wire for an externalization wire (after intubating the antegrade guide with the crossing wire or before snaring)
3. Externalizing the wire and attaching the antegrade copilot system
4. Treatment of the lesion, including ballooning and stenting
5. Removal of the externalization wire with active guide management and careful attention to preservation of the coronary ostium.

The Hybrid Approach for Percutaneous Revascularization of Coronary Chronic Total Occlusions

Craig A. Thompson, MD, MMSc

KEYWORDS

- Chronic total occlusion • Percutaneous coronary intervention • Coronary artery disease
- Left anterior descending coronary artery • Left circumflex coronary artery • Right coronary artery

KEY POINTS

- Percutaneous coronary intervention (PCI) for coronary chronic total occlusion (CTO) has been limited historically by poor success rates and clinical uptake.
- The hybrid approach for CTO PCI is based on an algorithm that is intended to create a process whereby trained operators react to angiograms and craft strategies in a similar manner.
- The goal of the hybrid approach is to combine technologies and techniques in a way that facilitates opportunities to attempt CTO PCI in patients with appropriate clinical indications irrespective of anatomy.
- Although PCI for CTO is rapidly evolving and these methods may be adapted over time, the hybrid approach can provide a starting point to expand the pool of operators.

INTRODUCTION

Successful percutaneous coronary intervention (PCI; see **Box 1** for other abbreviations used in this article) for coronary chronic total occlusion (CTO) in selected patients is associated with reduced mortality; improved angina, heart failure symptoms, and quality of life; and reduced need for subsequent coronary artery bypass surgery (CABG).[1,2] Despite ample evidence supporting promotion and education of this valuable therapy for patients, dissemination and uptake have been limited in broad clinical practice from the public health perspective.[3] This limited adoption is primarily attributable to technical difficulty of CTO PCI procedures and the common perception that the procedures, by their very nature, are prolonged and often unsuccessful. The consequence has been that most of these patients remain unrevascularized or are referred for open heart surgery.

The SYNTAX randomized trial CTO subset only had approximately 70% of CTOs revascularized in the surgical therapy arm, highlighting the fact that cardiac surgeons are also challenged by chronic occlusion. Often these targets are poor because of negative remodeling or diffuse disease, or location in positions difficult to adequately address (eg, atrioventricular groove of the LCx) despite an open chest. The end product is a situation in which some surgical and many medical patients are incompletely revascularized and subsequently have a large ischemic burden and/or severe lifestyle impairment. In addition, the "watch and wait" approach is complicated by

Conflicts of interest: Dr Thompson has consulting relationships with BridgePoint Medical, Abbott Vascular, and Terumo Medical Corporation, and has an equity position in BridgePoint Medical.
Cardiovascular Catheterization and Intervention, Yale New Haven Hospital, Yale University School of Medicine, 789 Howard Avenue, Dana 305, New Haven, CT 06517, USA
E-mail address: Craig.thompson@yale.edu

interventional.theclinics.com

poor physician judgment regarding symptoms, often with patients categorized as asymptomatic who in fact have severe impairment of quality of life. Specifically, many patients with coronary CTO do not experience typical angina. The symptom complex often more closely resembles diastolic heart failure syndrome, with complaints of dyspnea and fatigue. The patients may accommodate this insidious complex with reduction in activity and have subsequent severe life quality impairment. Although the optimal rate for appropriate CTO PCI is not well elucidated, the 11% to 13% national revascularization rate seen in the American College of Cardiology National Data Registry is clearly suboptimal.

CLASSIC TECHNIQUE AND THE MYTH OF THE TRUE LUMEN

Many operators have shown great historical, and current, interest in making efforts to heroic levels to "stay in the true lumen" when wiring the CTO segment. The primary cited reasons are a theoretic improvement in healing, a better safety-durability profile for drug-eluting stents placed during the procedure, and safety concerns when exploiting the subadventitial space as a treatment pathway. This author believes that the practical ramifications of this philosophy as a dogmatic approach are reduced success rates and prolonged procedures. Furthermore, methodical wire technique is perhaps the most difficult of skill sets to teach and learn, and cannot resolve the issues of best approaches to highly complex anatomy. Both technique and technologies designed to cross the true lumen or provide subintimal return do not consistently work using that mechanism (intravascular ultrasound [IVUS] of wire only, true-to-true technique reveals subadventitial pathways ~30%–50% of the time). Therefore, if the end goal is to have more open arteries, and treat all patients irrespective of anatomy with appropriate indications, then it should be recognized that

singular strategies will not adequately serve the public need.

Physicians have a tendency to reflect to intellectual comfort zones in interventional cardiology. Management of CTO challenges these constructs in several ways. Technology and techniques in 2012 for optimal CTO PCI can be counterintuitive to standard PCI procedures. For example, crossing catheters or looped wires in the subadventitial space provides greater safety than standard wire techniques; retrograde methods can be safer and more effective in selected patients than a standard antegrade approach; and Ellis grades 1 to 3 perforations are typically dissections and do not constitute a safety hazard or stopping point for many procedures. Another construct is "the true lumen." One must recall vascular morphology and biology and classification of endothelial, intima, media, and adventitial layers and internal and external elastic membranes. Within a completely occluded segment, histopathologic survey often demonstrates destruction of the integrity of these layers, and possibly disconnection with standard nondiseased vascular biologic function.[4] The adventitia, with its strength and elasticity, is the only layer to provide security in the vessel structure. If one can accept a clinical utility model that two effective layers are present in CTO, the adventitia and the plaque, then therapeutic options abound and opportunities to effectively manage patients will increase accordingly. Finally, it should be recognized that negative remodeling occurs in these vessels, and many that are considered small or poor targets in fact will enlarge (~30%) over time with restoration of flow and can provide fine clinical results for the patient.

HYBRID APPROACH FOR CTO PCI

The remainder of this article summarizes the hybrid approach for CTO PCI.

Prerequisites to the Hybrid Technique

The requisite knowledge base and skill sets assumed include

- CTO wiring strategies (wire shaping, selection, characteristics, and handling)
- Antegrade dissection reentry (practically speaking, the Stingray technology (BridgePoint Medical, Minneapolis, MN), although IVUS-guided intralesional rewiring would be included in this category)[5,6]
- Retrograde techniques, including the reverse controlled antegrade and retrograde tracking (reverse CART) and CART methods.[7–14]

These techniques have been described in detail elsewhere, so the nuances are omitted in this article to highlight practical application of the hybrid technique: "what to do when." During the learning phase, it is appropriate to leverage experience in a given strategy when technique overlap exists and net safety is neutral. The initial experiences with the more advanced strategies, such as dissection-reentry and retrograde methods, are best suited for new operators and programs that have an experienced proctor onsite in an advisory capacity. Proctors can be identified at national/regional training programs and also at www.cto fundamentals.org.

The Hybrid Approach for CTO PCI

The goal of the hybrid approach is to combine technologies and techniques in a manner that facilitates opportunities to attempt CTO PCI in patients with appropriate clinical indications irrespective of anatomy. The technical merits and emphasis are on procedural success and, importantly, procedural efficiency with an acceptable safety profile.[15] Efficient procedures and a process can help drive CTO PCI adoption (and therefore lead to primary initiative of more open arteries) and likely reduce complications specific to better management of radiation and contrast exposure, and perhaps reduce bleeding/thrombotic complications that have higher frequency rates in prolonged cases.

Hybrid CTO PCI refers to

1. A standard, simplified process to approach CTO PCI based on anatomy
2. Harmonizing antegrade and retrograde techniques
3. Harmonizing lesion wire- or device-based crossing with dissection-reentry methods.

Hybrid CTO PCI exploits the phenomenon of conditional probability and attempts to use high reward strategies at a point in the procedure that they are most likely to be successful, and endorses rapid change to alternative methods when failure modes dictate that secondary and bailout strategies have more probable positive outcome than the current strategy.

Anatomy Dictates Strategy

The initial angiogram is reviewed and an initial strategy, with provisional strategies, is developed before beginning the procedure (**Fig. 1**). Occasionally, additional angiography with the second catheter is required to completely inform this decision. Virtually all CTO PCI procedures with contralateral or multiple collateral beds should have the second catheter (a guide catheter if any possibility for retrograde exists) for optimal imaging. One should remember that collateral patterns often shift during the course of these procedures.

Four variables are considered:

1. Ambiguity of the proximal cap (can the proximal CTO cap be clearly identified with angiography or through use of an IVUS catheter in a nearby sidebranch)
2. Lesion length of 20 mm or more (longer lesions can be successfully wired with standard techniques, but success rates dramatically decline at this point and case times are prolonged)[16]
3. Quality of the distal target (size, imaging, degree of disease, and sidebranches of clinical interest)
4. Interventional collaterals (perceived likelihood of successful crossing of collaterals to use retrograde techniques in a safe and efficient manner).

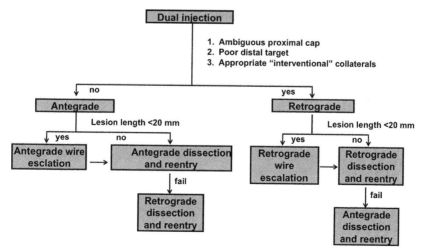

Fig. 1. The hybrid algorithm for CTO PCI based on initial angiogram results.

Based on these results, initial strategy is determined:

1. Antegrade, wire escalation: clear proximal cap, short lesion less than 20 mm, good target, interventional collaterals irrelevant
2. Antegrade dissection reentry: clear proximal cap, long lesion, good target, interventional collaterals irrelevant
3. Retrograde, wire escalation: ambiguous proximal cap, short lesion, good or poor target, suitable interventional collaterals
4. Retrograde dissection reentry: ambiguous proximal cap, long lesion, good or poor target, suitable interventional collaterals.

One should note that the driver for the primary retrograde technique, in order of relevance, is ambiguity of the proximal cap and poor target in patients with suitable collaterals. Nuanced methods to troubleshoot patients not in these anatomic bins exist, but are outside the scope of this article.

Secondary strategies are developed in advance in anticipation of failed or failing primary strategies. Generally, the secondary strategy for antegrade or retrograde wire escalation is the dissection-reentry method in the same direction. One should remember that the initial directional choice was determined by characteristics favoring success and efficiency with that direction (antegrade vs retrograde). Failed dissection reentry in one direction favors dissection reentry in the other direction as secondary or the final bailout strategy (eg, for failed dissection reentry antegrade, one should go retrograde and use reverse CART; for failed retrograde techniques, one should go antegrade with intent for Stingray reentry).

The "toolkit" for this approach is previously described in articles addressing the specific techniques used,[6,7,9,15] but includes:

- Wires:
  - Soft, tapered, polymer-jacketed wire for lesion probing and knuckle wire techniques (eg, Fiedler XT, Asahi Intecc Co., Ltd., Santa Ana, CA, USA)
  - Soft, nontapered, polymer-jacketed or hydrophilic wire for retrograde collateral crossing and lesion probing (eg, Fiedler FC and Asahi Sion, Asahi Intecc Co., Ltd.; Pilot 50, Abbott Vascular, Abbott Park, IL, USA)
  - Stiff polymer-jacketed wire for complex lesion wiring, dissection reentry, and knuckle wire technique (eg, Pilot 200, Abbott Vascular)
  - Stiff tapered wire for lesion penetration (eg, Confianza Pro 12 g, Abbott Vascular)
- Antegrade reentry tools:
  - Stingray Orienting Balloon and Stingray Guidewire (BridgePoint Medical)
- Retrograde tools:
  - Corsair Microcatheter (Asahi Intecc, Co., Ltd.)

In addition, other devices useful in CTO PCI but not specific to the hybrid approach include the GuideLiner Catheter (Vascular Solutions, Inc., Minneapolis, MN, USA), Tornus Microcatheter (Asahi Intecc Co., Ltd.), large and small snares, covered stents, and coils.

SUMMARY

Coronary CTO PCI has been limited historically by poor success rates and clinical uptake. Recent technique and technology advances have provided a platform to create a systematic method to improve success rates and efficiency and, importantly, to extend therapy to a broader group of patients with need, through addressing consistency and training needs and overcoming anatomic hurdles. This process is summarized in this article by the method known as hybrid CTO PCI. Although CTO PCI is rapidly evolving and these methods may, in turn, adapt over time, this method can provide a starting point to expand the pool of operators and, ideally, achieve the goal of "more open arteries" worldwide.

REFERENCES

1. Joyal D, Afilalo J, Rinfret S. Effectiveness of recanalization of chronic total occlusions: a systematic review and meta-analysis. Am Heart J 2010;160: 179–87.
2. Grantham JA, Jones PG, Cannon L, et al. Quantifying the early health status benefits of successful chronic total occlusion recanalization: results from the Flowcardia's Approach to Chronic Total Occlusion Recanalization (FACTOR) trial. Circ Cardiovasc Qual Outcomes 2010;3:284–90.
3. Grantham JA, Marso SP, Spertus J, et al. Chronic total occlusion angioplasty in the United States. JACC Cardiovasc Interv 2009;2:479–86.
4. Sumitsuji S, Inoue K, Ochiai M, et al. Fundamental wire technique and current standard strategy of percutaneous intervention for chronic total occlusion with histopathological insights. JACC Cardiovasc Interv 2011;4:941–51.
5. Whitlow PL, Burke MN, Lombardi WL, et al. Use of a novel crossing and re-entry system in coronary chronic total occlusions that have failed standard crossing techniques: results of the FAST-CTOs

(Facilitated Antegrade Steering Technique in Chronic Total Occlusions) trial. JACC Cardiovasc Interv 2012;5:393–401.

6. Whitlow PL, Lombardi WL, Araya M, et al. Initial experience with a dedicated coronary re-entry device for revascularization of chronic total occlusions. Catheter Cardiovasc Interv 2011. DOI: 10.1002/ccd.23417. [Epub ahead of print].

7. Brilakis ES, Grantham JA, Thompson CA, et al. The retrograde approach to coronary artery chronic total occlusions: a practical approach. Catheter Cardiovasc Interv 2012;79:3–19.

8. Jones DA, Weerackody R, Rathod K, et al. Successful recanalization of chronic total occlusions is associated with improved long-term survival. JACC Cardiovasc Interv 2012;5:380–8.

9. Joyal D, Thompson CA, Grantham JA, et al. The retrograde technique for recanalization of chronic total occlusions: a step-by-step approach. JACC Cardiovasc Interv 2012;5:1–11.

10. Thompson CA, Jayne JE, Robb JF, et al. Retrograde techniques and the impact of operator volume on percutaneous intervention for coronary chronic total occlusions an early U.S. experience. JACC Cardiovasc Interv 2009;2:834–42.

11. Kimura M, Katoh O, Tsuchikane E, et al. The efficacy of a bilateral approach for treating lesions with chronic total occlusions the CART (controlled antegrade and retrograde subintimal tracking) registry. JACC Cardiovasc Interv 2009;2:1135–41.

12. Rathore S, Katoh O, Matsuo H, et al. Retrograde percutaneous recanalization of chronic total occlusion of the coronary arteries: procedural outcomes and predictors of success in contemporary practice. Circ Cardiovasc Interv 2009;2:124–32.

13. Rathore S, Matsuo H, Terashima M, et al. Procedural and in-hospital outcomes after percutaneous coronary intervention for chronic total occlusions of coronary arteries 2002 to 2008: impact of novel guidewire techniques. JACC Cardiovasc Interv 2009;2:489–97.

14. Surmely JF, Tsuchikane E, Katoh O, et al. New concept for CTO recanalization using controlled antegrade and retrograde subintimal tracking: the CART technique. J Invasive Cardiol 2006;18:334–8.

15. Brilakis ES, Grantham JA, Rinfret S, et al. A percutaneous treatment algorithm for crossing coronary chronic total occlusions. JACC Cardiovasc Interv 2012;5:367–79.

16. Morino Y, Abe M, Morimoto T, et al. Predicting successful guidewire crossing through chronic total occlusion of native coronary lesions within 30 minutes: the J-CTO (Multicenter CTO Registry in Japan) score as a difficulty grading and time assessment tool. JACC Cardiovasc Interv 2011;4:213–21.

Transradial Approach for Chronic Total Occlusion Percutaneous Coronary Intervention

Rodrigo Bagur, MD, Stéphane Rinfret, MD, SM, FRCP(C)*

KEYWORDS

- Chronic total occlusion • Transradial • Percutaneous coronary intervention • Recanalization
- Bleeding

KEY POINTS

- The transradial approach has an important role in interventional cardiology.
- Bleeding complications have been recognized as powerful adverse predictors of subsequent mortality after percutaneous coronary intervention.
- The transradial approach has emerged as one of the effective bleeding prevention strategies.
- Chronic total occlusion (CTO) recanalization is likely to provide significant clinical benefits, even from a mortality standpoint.
- Transradial approach commit the operator to the use of smaller guide catheters, and this might be a concern when planning a complex PCI procedure such as CTO recanalization; however, experienced transradial operators have learned to overcome such limitations within the CTO recanalization scenario.

INTRODUCTION

Although chronic total occlusion (CTO) recanalization is likely to provide significant clinical benefits, even from a mortality standpoint,[1] no randomized trial has demonstrated such benefit compared with a planned optimal medical therapy strategy. Therefore, CTO remains under scrutiny from the interventional world.

Bleeding complications have been recognized as powerful adverse predictors of subsequent mortality after percutaneous coronary intervention (PCI); therefore, strategies to reduce such complications are likely to provide further benefits to patients. Among those bleeding prevention strategies, the transradial approach has emerged as a very effective one, to the point that an increasing

number of operators think this approach has value for many indications, including primary PCI for ST elevation myocardial infarction.[2–7] In many centers around the world, the transradial approach has largely replaced the transfemoral approach, to the point that some operators may be reluctant in performing CTO PCI because many experienced CTO operators have advocated the use of large 8F catheters to achieve success.

The radial approach has come a long way since its initial description, in 1989, by Campeau[8] for coronary angiography. Later, Kiemeneij and Laarman[9] reported its use for percutaneous coronary balloon angioplasty. Then, Kiemeneij and colleagues[10] investigated its use for stent implantation. From that time, the transradial approach has continued to gain a substantial role in interventional

Disclosures: The authors have nothing to disclose regarding the content of this manuscript.
Interventional Cardiology Laboratories, Quebec Heart & Lung Institute—Laval University, 2725 Chemin Sainte-Foy, G1V 4G5, Québec (Québec), Canada
* Corresponding author.
E-mail address: stephane.rinfret@criucpq.ulaval.ca

Intervent Cardiol Clin 1 (2012) 355–363
doi:10.1016/j.iccl.2012.03.003
2211-7458/12/$ – see front matter © 2012 Elsevier Inc. All rights reserved.

cardiology. In fact, a large body of evidence now supports the safety and feasibility of transradial approach in a broad spectrum of patients and settings. The spectrum ranges from diagnostic catheterization and staged PCI to ad-hoc PCI in acute coronary syndromes and primary PCI for ST-elevation myocardial infarction. Moreover, for complex PCI, such as unprotected left main PCI, saphenous vein graft PCI and, more recently, for CTO recanalization—even when involving the retrograde approach.[2–6,11–19]

Aside from bleeding reduction, patients undergoing transradial procedures have reported strong preference for the wrist approach because of prompt ambulation and comfort, leading to an improvement in their quality of life soon after the procedure.[20] Also, transradial approach allows for early discharge and, therefore, saves hospital costs.[21] However, in most situations, a transradial approach commits the operator to the use of smaller guide catheters,[5] which is often perceived to be a strong limitation by transfemoral PCI supporters, especially when contemplating a very complex PCI procedure such as CTO recanalization. Experienced transradial operators have learned to overcome such limitations in many situations. This article provides an overview of basic principles and techniques required to perform transradial CTO PCI.

GENERAL CONSIDERATIONS

Several studies have shown that the transradial approach, when compared with the transfemoral route, is associated with fewer access site bleeding complications and improved clinical outcomes, especially in patients with maximal platelet inhibition and/or anticoagulation therapies.[2–5,14,22] Femoral artery access has been traditionally advocated for CTO PCI by most interventional cardiologists because it allows for a broader use of 7F or 8F guide catheters. Large-bore catheters are known to provide better passive support and allow for the use of more equipment in the same guide. Therefore, in most series published on CTO PCI, the use of the femoral approach was largely preferred.[23–25]

However, in most cases of CTO PCI, considering the need for a dual arterial access, even when using contralateral guidance without a retrograde approach, using large catheters probably and logically doubles the risk of access site complication compared with a single arterial access.

Experienced transradial operators have recently reported their favorable experience, mitigating concerns about the effectiveness of the use of transradial approach and smaller catheters for CTO PCI and suggesting extremely safe outcomes, especially regarding bleeding and vascular issues. Kim and colleagues[15] first suggested the feasibility of the transradial approach for CTO PCI, whereas Taketani and colleagues[16] reported the first four cases of retrograde CTO recanalization using bilateral radial access. More recently, these results were echoed by Wu and colleagues,[17] Egred,[19] and Rinfret (coauthor of this article) and colleagues[18] in the early Canadian CTO recanalization experience.

Patient Set-up and Site Access

In the authors' center, which almost exclusively uses the transradial approach in more than 8000 diagnostic catheterizations and 3300 PCI yearly, the assessment of the deep palmar arch is routinely performed on both sides with plethysmography.[26] Both radial artery punctures are performed 1 to 2 cm above the styloid process by the traditional Seldinger technique.[27] Therefore, we prefer to transfix the posterior arterial wall by using a regular 18-G × 1 ¼ in (short) IV sheath (BD Insyte Autoguard, Mississauga, ON, Canada). After removing the needle, the IV sheath is pulled back up to the point of getting back-blood flow. At this point, we advance a short 0.035 in straight guidewire or a Bentson (Cook Medical, Bloomington, IN, USA) 0.035 in guidewire into the radial artery lumen. Following the insertion of a regular (non–hydrophilic-coated) short 6F or 7F introducer (as used for the femoral access), 2.5 mg verapamil is administered through the sheath. The left arm is then brought over the patient's abdomen and the left hand strapped to keep the left wrist toward the pubis, to improve patient and operator comfort (**Fig. 1**). The operator should never have to bend over the patient to reach the left radial access site; it is a matter of taking the time to properly position the patient. Then, the left radial access is used for the right coronary artery (RCA) catheter and the right radial access for the left coronary catheter to optimize support, no matter where the CTO is (in the left system or in the RCA). Although the right radial best serves for both coronary ostia, the authors strongly believe that optimal support is gained using a right radial for the left main guide instead of from a left radial. Importantly, for selected patients in which larger (≥7F) introducers or catheters are planned to be inserted, and based on the concept that the inner luminal diameter of the radial artery is usually smaller near the wrist,[28,29] an alternative is to perform the radial puncture a bit "higher" than usual; hence, puncturing between 5 to 7 cm above the styloid process, when appropriate. However,

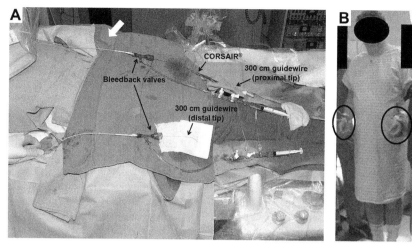

Fig. 1. Transradial CTO recanalization patient setup. (*A*) Patient over the table, two introducers are placed for the biradial access; the left arm (*white arrow*) is strapped to improve patient's comfort. (*B*) Patient stand up immediately after transradial CTO PCI (*black circles* highlight the hemostatic bracelets).

the authors strongly believe that 6F guides easily provide enough support for the retrograde side, in the Corsair (Asahi Intecc Co, Ltd, Japan) channel dilator era.

GUIDE CATHETER SIZE AND CURVE SELECTION

Guide catheter support and inner lumen size have been of some concern for CTO PCI. As a result, some interventional cardiologists, even when experienced with the radial approach for non–CTO PCI, would rather avoid the transradial route when planning CTO recanalization. However, to maximize guide inner-lumen size without compromising outer diameter at the wrist lever, 7.5F sheathless guides (Eau-Cath Sheathless, Asahi Intecc) may be considered from the radial approach, especially when trapping balloon technique may be frequently required, as with the use of the CrossBoss or StingRay (BridgePoint Medical, Plymouth, MN, USA) devices.[30,31] The 7.5F catheter has an external diameter of 2.49 mm, which is smaller than the external diameter of a conventional 6F introducer sheath (2.62 mm). However, the applicability of sheathless guide catheters for CTO recanalization is still largely unknown and embryonic; many operators have experienced reduced support in some situations using those hydrophilic-coated guides. It is noteworthy that larger bore regular guide catheters can also be used safely in selected cases. Several investigators have reported that 7F and, even, 8F catheters can be used through the radial artery, even with an introducer.[5,15–19,28,32] Thus, up to now, there is no standard rule regarding

the selection of guide catheters that should or should not be used for transradial CTO PCI. The authors, therefore, think that experienced transradial operators would prefer similar guide catheter shapes and size over conventional PCI in their daily practice. Therefore, the selection of a guide catheter has to be done based on the lesion characteristics and the patient's ascending aorta and radial artery size. Commonly, a 6F (7F, if needed) guide catheter may be the first choice. In fact, it has been demonstrated that 8F guide catheters are not mandatory for successful retrograde CTO recanalization.[18,33] Moreover, the authors strongly believe that the use of 6F guide catheters from the retrograde approach provides enough support for the advancement of the Corsair (Asahi Intecc) channel dilator and can be safely used. It may also improve procedure safety because smaller catheters probably reduce the risk for potential donor artery dissection, a feared complication when using the retrograde approach.[18,34] For RCA CTO intervention, the authors prefer Amplatz Left (AL) 0.75 or 1 curves, followed by Judkins Right (JR) 4 when minimal disease is present in the proximal segment, allowing for deep intubation if needed. In cases where the RCA exhibits some disease in the proximal or ostial portions, the use of a guide catheter with side holes reduces the risk of hydraulic dissection and allows for a more stable pressure curve assessment. When the RCA guide is the retrograde guide, the same curves may be selected, although 6F guide catheters are almost exclusively used, as previously explained. However, side holes should be avoided on the retrograde side because dampening of the retrograde pressure is extremely helpful information to guide catheter maneuvers to reduce donor artery problems. For left anterior descending CTO PCI, the authors prefer Extra Back-up (XB or EBU) 3.5 and, sometimes, 4.0 or 3.0 curves, depending on the size of the aortic root. For a left circumflex artery CTO PCI, AL2, or AL1 are preferred for coaxial orientation and optimal support, followed by XB curves. Use of 90-cm guide catheters, commercially available, is strongly advocated when a retrograde approach may be performed. Alternatively, to reduce inventory, shortening of the catheter can be done as published.[35,36] In addition, the COPILOT Bleedback control valve (Abbott Vascular) or its equivalent should be used on both guide catheters to reduce back bleeding during catheter manipulation, especially with devices that require rotation, such as the CrossBoss (BridgePoint Medical), the Corsair or the Tornus (Asahi Intecc).

Finally, although 5F catheters may be used from the contralateral side, especially when no retrograde approach is contemplated, the authors think that the current CTO therapies are better performed through larger guides, although this statement may change with future miniaturization of devices.

TECHNICAL CONSIDERATION WITH 6F GUIDE CATHETERS

It should be noted that Tornus (Asahi Intecc Co, Ltd, Japan) 2.1 mm or 2.6 mm devices, CrossBoss and Stingray catheters (BridgePoint Medical, Plymouth, MN, USA), as well as rotational atherectomy (up to a 1.5 mm burr) can be used in 6F guide catheters. When using the retrograde techniques, controlled antegrade and retrograde subintimal tracking (CART), reverse CART, or knuckle wire techniques can be effectively performed with 6F guides because most of the support is provided from the Corsair catheter inserted through the collateral channel—not from the guide catheter itself.

CLINICAL OUTCOMES AND PROCEDURAL COMPLICATIONS

In a series of 85 patients, Kim and colleagues[15] achieved a procedural success rate of 65.5%, using 6F guide catheters in most cases (81%). Only 6% of patients were switched to the femoral route because of guide catheter engagement failure, severe subclavian tortuosity or stenosis, radial artery loop, and/or poor guiding support. They reported no major access site complications.[15]

More recently, Wu and colleagues[17] showed that, for selected patients and lesions (in a series

of 85 patients) the transradial approach using even smaller (5F) guide catheters was feasible. The success rate was similar to that using a 6F catheter. However, most patients (91.4%) underwent CTO PCI through 6F guide catheters for the antegrade approach, while most (79%) retrograde procedures were performed with 7F guides.[17] Only minor access site complications (eg, forearm ecchymosis) were observed, in 3.5% of the patients.[17]

In the early Canadian transradial retrograde CTO PCI experience, Rinfret and colleagues[18] reported that 6F guides were used through bilateral transradial access in 88% of the patients, 71% from the antegrade side, and 91% from the retrograde side. This is a significant downsizing of guide size compared with the Wu and colleagues[17] series. With this approach, no access site bleeding or major vascular complications were noted.[18] In addition, the average hemoglobin drop from the morning before the procedure up to the next day after the procedure was only 0.75 ± 0.84 g/dL.[18] This very low hemoglobin drop and low vascular and bleeding complication rates were perceived to be the result of a preferred transradial approach over a femoral approach, the use of a 6F (or, rarely, 7F) guide catheters instead of 8F guide catheters, and the use of the COPILOT Bleedback valves instead of usual hemostatic valves.[18] Such a low bleeding complication rate is, therefore, expected to translate into better long-term clinical outcomes,[2,6,7,37–40] although studies comparing transfemoral to transradial CTO PCI are largely lacking.

In addition, data regarding catheter size, access site and ischemic complications are often underreported, which makes head-to-head comparisons even more difficult. Of note, Rathore and colleagues[12] reported on a large Japanese experience, including 468 patients, and compared the transradial (n = 318) and femoral (n = 150) approaches for CTO PCI. The success rates were similar for both approaches. Only 3.3% of the transradial patients were switched to the femoral approach because of radial artery spasm or anatomic variations in radial and subclavian arteries.[12] The procedural success rate in this comparison study was similar (>80%) to those shown in previous studies using the femoral approach. Not surprisingly, the overall access site complication rate was significantly higher in the femoral group (11.3% vs 3.5%). Minor access site complications among the femoral group occurred in 13 patients (8.7%) who developed small hematomas (<5 cm) or localized bruising that were managed conservatively. Only minor access site complications were related to the radial approach, including oozing, ecchymosis, and small hematoma (<2 cm) in 11 patients (3.5%).[12] All of these minor complications were managed conservatively with no impact on hospital discharge time. While four patients (2.7%) in the transfemoral group experienced large hematoma, including one with retroperitoneal extension that required blood transfusion, none of the transradial approach patients suffered from large hematoma. Of note, although 6F guide catheters were predominately used among the transradial group, 6F guide catheters were also used in 70%, 7F catheters in 18%, and 8F catheters in 12% of the patients treated from the femoral route.[12]

Fluoroscopy time and radiation exposure have been a major concern against the transradial approach for coronary PCI and thus hotly debated.[41,42] However, in light of the well-established advantages provided by the transradial access in terms of reducing bleeding and vascular complications,[22] the authors believe that such benefits can be applied to CTO PCI and largely mitigate any potential increase in radiation or contrast, which are driven by other non–site-related factors, such as complexity of the case, patient body size, and so forth. It should be highlighted that procedural and fluoroscopic times reported by Rathore and colleagues[12] in the comparison study of transradial versus transfemoral approaches for CTO recanalization were similar in both groups. Although 6F catheters may reduce amount of contrast load, Rathore and colleagues[12] showed no difference when comparing transradial versus transfemoral groups, although 70% of the transfemoral patients underwent CTO PCI using 6F guides.[12] On the other hand, the amount of contrast dye is expected to be higher among retrograde CTO recanalizations.[18,24,35] Use of a smaller guide from the retrograde side may reduce the contrast load, although it remains unproven at this time.

IMMEDIATE POSTPROCEDURAL CARE AND RECOVERY FOLLOWING TRANSRADIAL CTO PCI

Usually, on completion of the procedure, the radial arterial sheath is immediately removed on the table and hemostasis achieved by a hemostatic bracelet or other specific devices such as the Hemo-Stop (Zoom Co Medic, Quebec, Canada), Radistop (RADI, Uppsala, Sweden), and the TR Band (Terumo, Japan). In selected cases, patients can exit the catheterization laboratory by walking (see **Fig. 1**B) up to the recovery area, where they will stay for about 30 minutes. Following this initial observation period, they will be transferred to their rooms. Hemostatic

bracelets are left in place up to 2 hours following the procedure and removed once hemostasis is completed. For other non–CTO-transradial PCI, specific measures to reduce radial artery occlusion can be applied,[43,44] although the clinical impact, from the authors' perspective, is largely unknown. Radial occlusion remains asymptomatic in almost all patients, although it will preclude future use of the same access site. As mentioned, transradial access overcomes the limitations of femoral access by allowing earlier patient ambulation and reducing discomfort and bleeding issues. It is, thus, noteworthy that, on arrival to their room, patients are allowed to walk around, go to the bathroom, and even walk through the corridors, which is often perceived by patients and their family to be of great value.

Although the authors' center currently practices same-day discharge following uncomplicated transradial PCI, patients who undergo CTO PCI will usually remain hospitalized overnight after their procedure and be discharged the next day, unless the procedure was relatively simple (antegrade approach, with true-to-true passage, without immediate complication or perforation).

LIMITATIONS OF THE TRANSRADIAL APPROACH FOR CTO PCI
Access-Related Limitations

First, potential anatomic variations, such as high radial bifurcation, looping, small accessory radial arteries, subclavian-brachiocephalic tortuosity, buckling of the innominate artery, unfolded aorta with large aortic root, and retroesophageal aorta (also called artery lusoria) are the most common limitations to get access into the ascending aorta-coronary ostia.[45,46] When using two radials, the risk of encountering such anomalies is probably at least doubled. Having said that, one catheter can be inserted from the femoral approach in case of failed radial cannulation or access. As a result, the authors always prepare both groins for such, or for the unlikely event of the need for balloon pump support.

Guide Catheter Support-Related Limitations

Back-up support is a legitimate concern with CTO recanalization. Therefore, use of curves that provide the maximum passive support is advocated. For example, use of Judkins Left 4 should be discouraged. Other strategies can be used to improve support, even through 6F guides. The balloon anchoring technique can be used to gain extra guide catheter support by inflating a rapid-exchange balloon in a non–target vessel and holding its shaft with backward force while advancing another rapid-exchange balloon or stent to cross the target lesion.[47,48]

Deep coronary intubation ($\geq$20 mm into the vessel) with a guide catheter can also be undertaken in cases of balloon or stent delivery failure in the presence of calcified and/or tortuous arteries, although proximal disease, if present, usually needs to be addressed with balloon angioplasty or even stenting.[49–51] This technique has recently been complemented by "mother-in-child" catheters (Heartrail, Terumo, Japan, or the GuideLiner, Vascular Solutions Inc, Minneapolis, MN, USA). The Heartrail is a 5F catheter, 120 cm long (20 cm longer than standard catheters); therefore, it protrudes distally.[52–55] The GuideLiner catheter extension system is a rapid-exchange 20 cm soft catheter that is advanced into the guide catheter beyond the distal tip of the guide catheter to increase backup support in cases of complex PCI.[56]

Guide Catheter Size-Related Limitations

Another important issue is the limited space in 6F guide catheters, although it is almost never an issue from the retrograde side. To overcome those limitations in specific situations, it is preferable to use a sheathless 7.5F guide from the antegrade side, although it is currently not available in the United States. These guides allow for almost all maneuvers that can usually only be performed through 8F guides. One especially useful technique in CTO PCI is the use of trapping wire.[57] It is currently not possible to use the trapping technique with a monorail balloon on a short 180 cm CTO guidewire while advancing a Tornus 2.6, a Corsair, a CrossBoss catheter, a StingRay balloon, or even most over-the-wire balloons. Therefore, traditional over-the-wire exchange using a 300 cm guidewire or an extension will often be required in 6F catheters. It is also impossible to perform intravascular ultrasound (IVUS)-guided proximal cap puncture through a 6F catheter using a microcatheter and a 5F-compatible Volcano Eagle Eye Gold Catheter (Volcano Therapeutics, Rancho Cordova, CA, USA).

However, all the aforementioned techniques can be easily performed through 7.5F sheathless guides. Finally, it is important to remember that only 7F-compatible covered stents are available in the United States (whereas 6F-compatible covered stents are available in Europe, Japan, or Canada). Such issues should be considered when selecting the antegrade guide size.

It is nevertheless possible and safe to perform most CTO PCI with the use of 6F guides.[18] Here is a list of the maneuvers that can still be

Table 1		
What can or cannot be performed with 6F guide catheters		
	YES	NO
Trapping wire and Tornus 2.1 mm	X	
Trapping wire and Tornus 2.6 mm		X
Trapping wire and Corsair		X
Trapping wire and FineCross	X	
Deep intubation	X	
Anchoring balloon technique with 1 monorail balloon and Tornus 2.1 mm, or one other monorail balloon	X	
Kissing balloon inflation using 2 monorail balloons or 1 stent delivery system and 1 monorail balloon	X	
IVUS-guided proximal cap puncture with microcatheter in place		X

performed through 6F: (1) trapping balloon technique and FineCross in the same guide, (2) trapping balloon technique and Tornus 2.1, and (3) kissing balloon inflation or anchoring balloon technique using two monorail (or rapid-exchange) balloons. Attention should be paid on the size of the monorail balloon shaft to be used; the smallest shafts provide better performance and reduce subsequent material interaction. Finally, although an IVUS probe cannot be used with a microcatheter at the same time, IVUS can be performed through 6F catheters as long it is the only device used in the guide. Moreover, IVUS-guided proximal cap puncture can be performed through a 6F catheter only if a CTO guidewire is used and not with a microcatheter. **Table 1** summarizes what can or cannot be done through a 6F guide catheter for transradial CTO PCI.

SUMMARY

Initial experience with the transradial approach for CTO PCI, even when bilateral, shows that it is feasible, teachable, and probably safer because it substantially reduces the risk of major access site bleeding complications. By committing to the use of smaller guides, transradial CTO PCI has some disadvantages that can, however, be mitigated by a better understanding of 6F-compatible CTO techniques.

REFERENCES

1. Joyal D, Afilalo J, Rinfret S. Effectiveness of recanalization of chronic total occlusions: a systematic

review and meta-analysis. Am Heart J 2010;160(1):179–87.

2. Mann T, Cubeddu G, Bowen J, et al. Stenting in acute coronary syndromes: a comparison of radial versus femoral access sites. J Am Coll Cardiol 1998;32(3):572–6.

3. Agostoni P, Biondi-Zoccai GG, de Benedictis ML, et al. Radial versus femoral approach for percutaneous coronary diagnostic and interventional procedures; systematic overview and meta-analysis of randomized trials. J Am Coll Cardiol 2004;44(2):349–56.

4. Rao SV, Ou FS, Wang TY, et al. Trends in the prevalence and outcomes of radial and femoral approaches to percutaneous coronary intervention: a report from the National Cardiovascular Data Registry. JACC Cardiovasc Interv 2008;1(4):379–86.

5. Bertrand OF, Rao SV, Pancholy S, et al. Transradial approach for coronary angiography and interventions: results of the first international transradial practice survey. JACC Cardiovasc Interv 2010;3(10):1022–31.

6. Jolly SS, Yusuf S, Cairns J, et al. Radial versus femoral access for coronary angiography and intervention in patients with acute coronary syndromes (RIVAL): a randomised, parallel group, multicentre trial. Lancet 2011;377(9775):1409–20.

7. Mamas MA, Ratib K, Routledge H, et al. Influence of access site selection on PCI-related adverse events in patients with STEMI: meta-analysis of randomised controlled trials. Heart 2012;98(4):303–11.

8. Campeau L. Percutaneous radial artery approach for coronary angiography. Cathet Cardiovasc Diagn 1989;16(1):3–7.

9. Kiemeneij F, Laarman GJ. Percutaneous transradial artery approach for coronary stent implantation. Cathet Cardiovasc Diagn 1993;30(2):173–8.

10. Kiemeneij F, Laarman GJ, de Melker E. Transradial artery coronary angioplasty. Am Heart J 1995;129(1):1–7.

11. Burzotta F, Trani C, Hamon M, et al. Transradial approach for coronary angiography and interventions in patients with coronary bypass grafts: tips and tricks. Catheter Cardiovasc Interv 2008;72(2):263–72.

12. Rathore S, Hakeem A, Pauriah M, et al. A comparison of the transradial and the transfemoral approach in chronic total occlusion percutaneous coronary intervention. Catheter Cardiovasc Interv 2009;73(7):883–7.

13. Rathore S, Roberts E, Hakeem AR, et al. The feasibility of percutaneous transradial coronary intervention for saphenous vein graft lesions and comparison with transfemoral route. J Interv Cardiol 2009;22(4):336–40.

14. Caputo RP, Tremmel JA, Rao S, et al. Transradial arterial access for coronary and peripheral procedures: executive summary by the transradial committee of the SCAI. Catheter Cardiovasc Interv 2011;78(6):823–39.

15. Kim JY, Lee SH, Choe HM, et al. The feasibility of percutaneous transradial coronary intervention for chronic total occlusion. Yonsei Med J 2006;47(5):680–7.

16. Taketani Y, Kaneda H, Saito S. Successful coronary intervention for chronic total occlusion using a retrograde approach with biradial arteries. J Invasive Cardiol 2007;19(9):E281–4.

17. Wu CJ, Fang HY, Cheng CI, et al. The safety and feasibility of bilateral radial approach in chronic total occlusion percutaneous coronary intervention. Int Heart J 2011;52(3):131–8.

18. Rinfret S, Joyal D, Nguyen CM, et al. Retrograde recanalization of chronic total occlusions from the transradial approach; early Canadian experience. Catheter Cardiovasc Interv 2011;78(3):366–74.

19. Egred M. Feasibility and safety of 7-Fr radial approach for complex PCI. J Interv Cardiol 2011;24(5):383–8.

20. Cooper CJ, El-Shiekh RA, Cohen DJ, et al. Effect of transradial access on quality of life and cost of cardiac catheterization: a randomized comparison. Am Heart J 1999;138(3 Pt 1):430–6.

21. Rinfret S, Kennedy WA, Lachaine J, et al. Economic impact of same-day home discharge after uncomplicated transradial percutaneous coronary intervention and bolus-only abciximab regimen. JACC Cardiovasc Interv 2010;3(10):1011–9.

22. Jolly SS, Amlani S, Hamon M, et al. Radial versus femoral access for coronary angiography or intervention and the impact on major bleeding and ischemic events: a systematic review and meta-analysis of randomized trials. Am Heart J 2009;157(1):132–40.

23. Morino Y, Kimura T, Hayashi Y, et al. In-hospital outcomes of contemporary percutaneous coronary intervention in patients with chronic total occlusion insights from the J-CTO Registry (Multicenter CTO Registry in Japan). JACC Cardiovasc Interv 2010;3(2):143–51.

24. Thompson CA, Jayne JE, Robb JF, et al. Retrograde techniques and the impact of operator volume on percutaneous intervention for coronary chronic total occlusions an early U.S. experience. JACC Cardiovasc Interv 2009;2(9):834–42.

25. Hsu JT, Tamai H, Kyo E, et al. Traditional antegrade approach versus combined antegrade and retrograde approach in the percutaneous treatment of coronary chronic total occlusions. Catheter Cardiovasc Interv 2009;74(4):555–63.

26. Barbeau GR, Arsenault F, Dugas L, et al. Evaluation of the ulnopalmar arterial arches with pulse oximetry and plethysmography: comparison with the

Allen's test in 1010 patients. Am Heart J 2004; 147(3):489–93.

27. Seldinger SI. Catheter replacement of the needle in percutaneous arteriography; a new technique. Acta Radiol 1953;39(5):368–76.

28. Saito S, Ikei H, Hosokawa G, et al. Influence of the ratio between radial artery inner diameter and sheath outer diameter on radial artery flow after transradial coronary intervention. Catheter Cardiovasc Interv 1999;46(2):173–8.

29. Fujii T, Masuda N, Toda E, et al. Analysis of right radial artery for transradial catheterization by quantitative angiography–anatomical consideration of optimal radial puncture point. J Invasive Cardiol 2010;22(8):372–6.

30. Mamas MA, Fath-Ordoubadi F, Fraser DG. Atraumatic complex transradial intervention using large bore sheathless guide catheter. Catheter Cardiovasc Interv 2008;72(3):357–64.

31. Mamas M, D'Souza S, Hendry C, et al. Use of the sheathless guide catheter during routine transradial percutaneous coronary intervention: a feasibility study. Catheter Cardiovasc Interv 2010;75(4): 596–602.

32. From AM, Gulati R, Prasad A, et al. Sheathless transradial intervention using standard guide catheters. Catheter Cardiovasc Interv 2010;76(7):911–6.

33. Fang HY, Wu CJ. Recanalization of calcified left anterior descending artery chronic total occlusion with rotational atherectomy via bilateral radial approach. Catheter Cardiovasc Interv 2011;78(6): 873–9.

34. Joyal D, Thompson CA, Grantham JA, et al. The retrograde technique for recanalization of chronic total occlusions: a step-by-step approach. JACC Cardiovasc Interv 2012;5(1):1–11.

35. Wu EB, Chan WW, Yu CM. Retrograde chronic total occlusion intervention: tips and tricks. Catheter Cardiovasc Interv 2008;72(6):806–14.

36. Kim TH, Jang Y. A new technique for shortening a guiding catheter during retrograde recanalization of a chronic total occlusion. Catheter Cardiovasc Interv 2011;77(3):358–62.

37. Manoukian SV, Voeltz MD, Eikelboom J. Bleeding complications in acute coronary syndromes and percutaneous coronary intervention: predictors, prognostic significance, and paradigms for reducing risk. Clin Cardiol 2007;30(10 Suppl 2): II24–34.

38. Feit F, Voeltz MD, Attubato MJ, et al. Predictors and impact of major hemorrhage on mortality following percutaneous coronary intervention from the REPLACE-2 Trial. Am J Cardiol 2007;100(9):1364–9.

39. Voeltz MD, Patel AD, Feit F, et al. Effect of anemia on hemorrhagic complications and mortality following percutaneous coronary intervention. Am J Cardiol 2007;99(11):1513–7.

40. Manoukian SV, Feit F, Mehran R, et al. Impact of major bleeding on 30-day mortality and clinical outcomes in patients with acute coronary syndromes: an analysis from the ACUITY Trial. J Am Coll Cardiol 2007;49(12):1362–8.

41. Lange HW, von Boetticher H. Randomized comparison of operator radiation exposure during coronary angiography and intervention by radial or femoral approach. Catheter Cardiovasc Interv 2006;67(1): 12–6.

42. Mercuri M, Mehta S, Xie C, et al. Radial artery access as a predictor of increased radiation exposure during a diagnostic cardiac catheterization procedure. JACC Cardiovasc Interv 2011;4(3): 347–52.

43. Pancholy S, Coppola J, Patel T, et al. Prevention of radial artery occlusion-patent hemostasis evaluation trial (PROPHET study): a randomized comparison of traditional versus patency documented hemostasis after transradial catheterization. Catheter Cardiovasc Interv 2008;72(3):335–40.

44. Plante S, Cantor WJ, Goldman L, et al. Comparison of bivalirudin versus heparin on radial artery occlusion after transradial catheterization. Catheter Cardiovasc Interv 2010;76(5):654–8.

45. Lo TS, Nolan J, Fountzopoulos E, et al. Radial artery anomaly and its influence on transradial coronary procedural outcome. Heart 2009;95(5):410–5.

46. Freestone B, Nolan J. Transradial cardiac procedures: the state of the art. Heart 2010;96(11): 883–91.

47. Hirokami M, Saito S, Muto H. Anchoring technique to improve guiding catheter support in coronary angioplasty of chronic total occlusions. Catheter Cardiovasc Interv 2006;67(3):366–71.

48. Lee NH, Suh J, Seo HS. Double anchoring balloon technique for recanalization of coronary chronic total occlusion by retrograde approach. Catheter Cardiovasc Interv 2009;73(6):791–4.

49. Peels HO, van Boven AJ, den Heijer P, et al. Deep seating of six French guiding catheters for delivery of new Palmaz-Schatz stents. Cathet Cardiovasc Diagn 1996;38(2):210–3.

50. Bartorelli AL, Lavarra F, Trabattoni D, et al. Successful stent delivery with deep seating of 6 French guiding catheters in difficult coronary anatomy. Catheter Cardiovasc Interv 1999;48(3): 279–84.

51. Abhaichand RK, Lefevre T, Louvard Y, et al. Amplatzing a 6 Fr Judkins right guiding catheter for increased success in complex right coronary artery anatomy. Catheter Cardiovasc Interv 2001;53(3): 405–9.

52. Takahashi S, Saito S, Tanaka S, et al. New method to increase a backup support of a 6 French guiding coronary catheter. Catheter Cardiovasc Interv 2004;63(4):452–6.

53. Mamas MA, Fath-Ordoubadi F, Fraser D. Successful use of the Heartrail III catheter as a stent delivery catheter following failure of conventional techniques. Catheter Cardiovasc Interv 2008;71(3):358–63.

54. Shaukat A, Al-Bustami M, Ong PJ. Chronic total occlusion—use of a 5 French guiding catheter in a 6 French guiding catheter. J Invasive Cardiol 2008;20(6):317–8.

55. Hayashida K, Louvard Y, Lefevre T. Transradial complex coronary interventions using a five-in-six system. Catheter Cardiovasc Interv 2011;77(1): 63–8.

56. Mamas MA, Fath-Ordoubadi F, Fraser DG. Distal stent delivery with Guideliner catheter: first in man experience. Catheter Cardiovasc Interv 2010;76(1): 102–11.

57. Ge JB, Zhang F, Ge L, et al. Wire trapping technique combined with retrograde approach for recanalization of chronic total occlusion. Chin Med J (Engl) 2008;121(17):1753–6.

Informed Consent of the Chronic Total Occlusion Patient

Evan Lau, MD, Patrick Whitlow, MD*

KEYWORDS

- Informed consent • Chronic total occlusion • Revascularization

KEY POINTS

- Informed consent is an important part of the preprocedural evaluation before a chronic total occlusion (CTO) intervention.
- The basic components of informed consent include descriptions of the nature of the procedure, risks, benefits, and alternatives.
- The overall success rate of a CTO intervention, which is lower than conventional coronary intervention, is a function of several factors, including lesion morphology and operator experience.
- Important risks to consider for CTO intervention include death, coronary perforation, radiation-induced skin injury, and contrast nephropathy.
- The primary benefits of CTO revascularization are angina relief and decrement of ischemic burden. Other potential benefits include improvement in left ventricular function and mortality; however, these are not universally accepted.

INTRODUCTION

Informed consent is becoming increasingly important in today's clinical practice, and its role in the interventional management of chronic total occlusions must be considered. In theory, patients should have a clear understanding of the benefits of any procedure they undergo, as well as the risks that are posed by the proposed procedure and the alternative treatment options. With this information, one can expect them to make informed decisions with regards to their medical care. In practice, there are many difficulties encountered in trying to achieve these ideals. The interventionalist must navigate the ambiguities of the legal and ethical standards of informed consent. This article will focus on the general principles of informed consent, then highlight the particular risks associated with chronic total occlusion (CTO) interventions. The goal of this article is to provide a basic framework for the interventional cardiologist to use when having consent discussions with his or her patients.

BACKGROUND

From a historical perspective, informed consent is a foreign concept to the medical field. The earliest medical traditions often warned against full disclosure to patients, believing that the patient's unyielding faith in the physician and therapeutic strategy was an essential part of recovery. There was a fear that disclosure of too much information could lead to poor decision making by the patient. The introduction of anxiety or doubt could be counterproductive to the patient's recovery. There was little faith in the patient's ability to understand his or her medical condition and make the medically correct decision. There was also a belief that the patient, in most circumstances, was unwilling to make decisions about his or her own medical care. The backbone of this traditional

Robert and Suzanne Tomsich Department of Cardiovascular Medicine, Cleveland Clinic Foundation, 9500 Euclid Avenue, Cleveland, OH 44118, USA
* Corresponding author.
E-mail address: whitlop@ccf.org

Intervent Cardiol Clin 1 (2012) 365–372
doi:10.1016/j.iccl.2012.04.005
2211-7458/12/$ – see front matter © 2012 Published by Elsevier Inc.

ideology is the benevolent physician, a sober agent who is able to decide and act in the best interest of the patient.

Current medical practice is shifting away from this paternalistic ideology of medicine. There is greater emphasis on patient autonomy and recognition of the patient's role in medical decision making. Several things are driving this paradigm shift. Controversy within the medical field often obscures the medically correct choice in a given clinical scenario. There is recognition that differences in an individual's values may lead to variability in choice of medical treatments, particularly invasive therapies that include significant risk. There is benefit from a legal perspective; apprising the patient of procedural risks and obtaining consent may help to avoid malpractice lawsuits, or at least protect the interventionalist in the case of a lawsuit.

Legal Evolution

The legal history of informed consent has evolved from case law dating back to the early 1900s. In Schloendorff v New York Hospital (1914), the obligation for patient consent to medical procedures was first established, based on the individual's right of self-determination. In Salgo v Leland Stanford, Jr. University Board of Trustees (1957), "informed" became an important part of obtaining a patient's consent. Although the details of the information to be disclosed were still ambiguous, the backbone of disclosure was established. The nature of the procedure and its consequences, risks and alternatives to the procedure must be discussed with and agreed upon by the patient. The extent of disclosure, particularly as it pertains to risk, continues to be a challenging and ambiguous area. In Canterbury v Spence (1972), the opinion given by the court stated that the content and amount of information should be enough for a patient to make an intelligent choice. The court still recognized that rational people may not make the same decision even if placed in similar circumstances.[1]

When examining the legal perspective of this issue, it is worth noting the legal concepts of battery versus negligence. When cases surrounding informed consent are tried, the courts may view the issue in 1 of these 2 legal concepts. For instance, in cases where there may have been inadequate demonstration of informed consent, deciding a case on the basis of battery places the burden on the physician for providing adequate disclosure, so that a patient can make an informed decision. In the absence of this, the procedure is seen as an intrusion on the part of the physician,

as priority is given to the patient's right to make decisions for his or her own treatment. Conversely, if the same case is decided on the basis of negligence, the physician is required to disclose as much as what a reasonable doctor would disclose. In this situation, the emphasis is not on the patient's self-determination, but rather that the physician has acted in accordance with standards of practice. As such, these cases involve the use of physician expert witnesses, with arguments attempting to establish what the standard of care would be. In contrast, the arguments made in battery cases do not necessarily require expert testimonial. Most cases pertaining to informed consent have been tried on the basis of negligence law, although more recent case law may involve viewing these cases with both concepts in mind.[2]

Elements of Informed Consent (Legal and Ethical Perspectives)

When deciding on the important elements of informed consent, one may consider both the ethical and legal perspectives. From an ethical standpoint, informed consent involves:

- Disclosure
- Comprehension
- Voluntariness
- Competence
- Consent.

In addition to the cardiologist's role in the process, namely disclosure, there is emphasis on the patient's ability to understand, process information, and consent to the procedure. In contrast, from a legal perspective, the focus is primarily on the content of information that the physician delivers:

- Nature of the procedure
- Risks
- Benefits
- Alternatives.

The challenge for the procedural cardiologist is to create a consenting process that is both efficient and comprehensive, as far as touching on all of these factors. Despite this framework, there remain ambiguities as far as the practical application of informed consent. In particular, how much information is required, particularly with respect to disclosure of risks. It is difficult to give specifics that would cover every situation, but several principles can be applied:

- As much information as would be required for a reasonable patient to make a decision

- As much information as a prudent physician would provide.

Even with these directives, it is difficult to determine exactly what risks one is required to disclose. It certainly is not practical or good for patient care to provide a litany of all possible complications that may occur. From a legal standpoint, it is likely sufficient to provide the most common and worst complications; it would follow that if a patient might be willing to accept those risks, he or she might be willing to accept a lesser or unforeseen complication should it occur. When enumerating the proposed benefits of a procedure and its alternatives, the interventionalist should consider a brief description of the evidence for the proposed benefits: whether it stems from anecdotal experience, clinical trial data or best, educated guess. If there is controversy in the field, that should be included in the discussion as well.[3]

NATURE OF THE PROCEDURE
Procedural Success

Published series show that the overall success rate of CTO interventions approach 70% to 80%.[4,5] Anatomic characteristics of the lesion will impact the likelihood of recanalization. Lesions that have been occluded for more than 3 months, are longer than 15 mm in length, have an abrupt (opposed to tapered) cut-off, and present with bridging collaterals portend an unfavorable prognosis for opening.[6] Operator experience is extremely important in determining the final outcome of these complex interventions. One study showed that high-volume CTO operators (≥75 CTO interventions) in the United States had a success rate of greater than 75%, as compared with lower volume operators (59% technical success rate). In addition, those operators with more experience tended to improve over time, with greater than 90% success rates, whereas their inexperienced counterparts did not change over time.[7] This suggests a rather slow, gradual learning curve.

Long-Term Outcomes

The use of drug-eluting stents has significantly decreased the overall rate of stent related complications in CTO interventions. The primary stenting of totally occluded native coronary arteries (PRISON) II study compared bare-metal stents (BMS) to sirolimus-eluting stent (SES). There was a significant reduction in major adverse cardiovascular endpoints (36% BMS group vs 12% SES over 3 years), driven largely by target vessel revascularization (**Fig. 1**). Binary in-segment restenosis rates were decreased from 41% in BMS versus 11% in SES. In this 1 study, the SES group demonstrated a 7% risk for stent thrombosis (definite and probable stent thrombosis events by the Academic Research Consortium definition).[8]

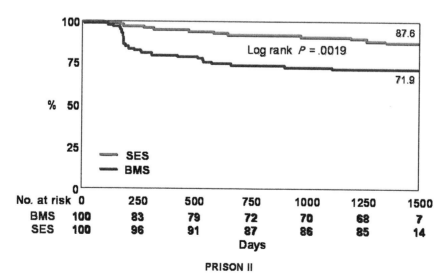

PRISON II

Fig. 1. Freedom from MACE (death, myocardial infarction, and TLR) in the PRISON II study. SES, sirolimus-eluting stent; BMS, bare-metal stent; MACE, major adverse cardiac event; TLR, target lesion revascularization. (*Adapted from* Rahel BM, Laarman GJ, Kelder JC, et al. Three-year clinical outcome after primary stenting of totally occluded native coronary arteries: a randomized comparison of bare-metal stent implantation with sirolimus-eluting stent implantation for the treatment of total coronary occlusions. Am Heart J 2009;157(1):149–55; with permission.)

RISKS

The following discussion will focus on complications that are specific for CTO cases. As stated previously, the process of consent should not degenerate into a litany of all possible complications, but rather the most severe complications, the possibility of which may alter the patient's consent, and procedurally specific complications that occur with relative frequency. One approach to addressing the first issue is to include the possibility of death or stroke when describing the risks of the procedure. Although the risk for these outcomes is exceedingly low, they are important considerations in the patient's personal calculation of whether to accept the risk of the procedure. If consent is obtained, the acknowledgment and acceptance of these risks may imply their acceptance of less severe complications also.

In the ensuing discussion, the authors will address the complications that are either specific to CTO interventions or occur with greater frequency than in other coronary cases.

Procedural Complications

The complexity of CTO intervention lends itself to a variety of procedural complications. Surprisingly, the latest published series of CTO interventions show that the procedural complication rate is low (**Table 1**). Across several series, the in-hospital death rate was 0.4% to 1.3%.[4,5,9] Postprocedural myocardial infarction rates ranged from 2% to 5%, and need for emergency CABG occurred in 0.7% of cases. Comparisons of CTO versus non-CTO interventions in matched cohorts show that the in-hospital complication rates are similar (**Fig. 2**). This is not to say that CTO interventions should be considered low-risk procedures. Whether the published complication rates apply to any

specific operator or a given case depends on operator experience and aggressiveness, as well as patient-specific anatomy. One of the most common and significant complications is that of coronary perforation, which was encountered in 7.2% of CTO interventions in 1 series. The majority of these perforations (71.4%) represented contrast staining alone, with resolution after observation only.[5] In this series, progression to tamponade occurred in 0.2% of cases; the Mayo Clinic experience showed a risk of tamponade of approximately 1%.[4,5]

In an antegrade approach, procedural risks include injury to the proximal vessel or side branches and vessel perforation during attempt to cross the CTO. If the CTO is crossed and wire placement in the true lumen is not confirmed, there is risk for closure of the distal artery if intervention is performed in a dissection plane. For a retrograde approach, a unique set of complications is possible. The donor vessel may be injured, dissected, or thrombosed in an attempt to cross a collateral vessel. Manipulation of the collateral vessel could cause closure and consequent ischemia to the CTO territory. Perforation of collateral channels is possible, as they are thin-walled structures. Epicardial collateral perforation may tend toward pericardial bleeding with resultant tamponade; these should never be dilated in hopes of passing equipment. In the case of septal collaterals, perforation may result in coronary fistulazation with a cardiac chamber, or development of an intramyocardial hematoma. The latter can usually be managed conservatively, but on occasion may require embolization to prevent expansion and worsening pain.

Radiation Injury

Radiation injury can be divided into 2 categories: deterministic and stochastic effects. Deterministic effects require a minimum number of cells to be injured before a biologic effect is seen; for instance, this includes hair loss and erythema. For these types of effects, a certain threshold dosage would guarantee a 100% likelihood of seeing that effect in a given patient. Stochastic effects relate to changes that may occur in a single cell, such as a mutation, that may ultimately lead to a biologic outcome. Although increasing dosage will increase the likelihood of seeing this effect, there are no threshold dosages that would guarantee that these effects occur. Stochastic effects include the development of malignancy following radiation exposure.

There is increasing concern for the stochastic effects of medical imaging, namely the relationship

Table 1 CTO PCI: major complications		
	JCTO (JACC Int 2010)	Mayo (03–05)
Death	0.4%	0
Emergency CABG	0.3%	0.7%
QMI	0.2%	3.3%
Non-QMI	2.1%	1.7%
Typical rate Death/CABG/ myocardial infarction	~4%–6%	

Abbreviations: JACC, Journal of American College of Cardiology; JCTO, Japanese Chronic Total Occlusion Club.

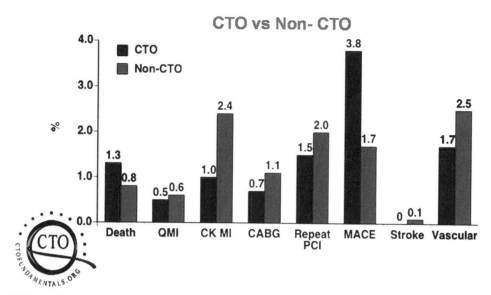

Fig. 2. Mid-America PCI complications. QMI, Q-wave myocardial infarction; CK MI, elevation in creatine kinase. (*Data from* Suero JA, Marso SP, Jones PG, et al. Procedural outcomes and long-term survival among patients undergoing percutaneous coronary intervention of a chronic total occlusion in native coronary arteries: a 20-year experience. J Am Coll Cardiol 2001;38(2):409–14; with permission.)

between malignancy and lifetime radiation exposure. Radiation doses associated with most medical imaging modalities do not achieve high enough thresholds to worry about the occurrence of deterministic effects.[10] CTO interventions require longer fluoroscopy times than single or multivessel interventions in non-occluded arteries, making deterministic radiation complications a real possibility. This results in radiation doses that can be 5 times higher than comparison interventions.[11] Generally speaking, skin changes can be seen in doses as low as 2 Gy, with desquamation occurring in 10 Gy to 15 Gy and necrosis at 18 Gy.[12] CTO interventions average 3.2 Gy, with some complex, long CTO interventions that easily exceed thresholds for serious skin injury. High radiation doses can be expected in long, complex cases, but also should be anticipated in obese patients. Exposure incurred during previous procedures should be taken into account and may warrant delay in initiating subsequent attempts at recanalization. Efforts should be made to minimize radiation exposure, including increased field of view, minimizing steepness of angulation, and using multiple working views to minimize exposure to a single field.

Contrast-Induced Nephropathy

The risk for contrast-induced nephropathy is primarily a function of the patient's baseline renal function and the contrast volume used during the procedure. Other variables, including age, heart failure, shock, diabetes mellitus, and others have also been associated with the development of nephropathy following coronary intervention.[13] That said, the modifiable variables, particularly in an elective situation, are the selection of patients who are at low risk (good baseline renal function) and minimization of contrast volume used. However, CTO interventions tend to be complex and often require a substantial amount of contrast volume for safe, procedural completion. In 1 case series of CTO interventions, the median contrast volume used, 293 mL (range 53–1097 mL), resulted in a 1.2% rate of contrast-induced nephropathy.[5] Traditionally, the maximal acceptable contrast dose is calculated at 5 mL contrast times body weight (kg)/serum creatinine (mg/dL). However, contrast-induced nephropathy has been reported to occur with use of volumes less than this amount. One criticism of this formula is that it does not account for a patient's age, which is a critical part of determining underlying renal function. A recent paper used calculated creatinine clearance to determine a safe contrast dose.[14] In that analysis, a procedural contrast volume of less than 2 times calculated creatinine clearance (mL/min) provided a reasonable discriminator of risk of nephropathy and requirement for dialysis, particularly in elective coronary intervention. One should take these contrast volume boundaries into account when determining the risk/benefit ratio of the procedure for an individual case.

BENEFITS
Angina Relief

One of the primary benefits of CTO recanalization is symptom relief and attenuation of ischemia. In observational cohorts of patients with successful versus unsuccessful recanalization of CTOs, there is a higher rate of freedom from angina (88.7% vs 75.0%) and improvement in exercise tolerance testing at 12 month follow-up.[15] CTO recanalization results in improvement in a number of subjective measures, including angina frequency, physical limitation, and overall quality of life.[16,17] In cohorts with successful CTO recanalization, there is a statistically significant improvement in Canadian Cardiovascular Society angina classification, with higher percentages of patients falling into the asymptomatic and class 1 angina categories.[18] This is accompanied by objective decrease in ischemic burden, particularly for those patients with 10% or greater ischemia as defined by nuclear perfusion imaging.[16] Another outcome worth considering is the rate of coronary artery bypass graft (CABG) in patients undergoing successful CTO percutaneous coronary intervention (PCI) versus those who have failed CTO interventions. Arguably, this is an important outcome from a patient's standpoint, as many people would consider avoidance of a life-changing surgery a valuable goal. Studies have demonstrated that there is a significant reduction in need for subsequent CABG in those patients undergoing successful CTO recanalization (3.2% vs 13.3% over 5 years).[19]

Left Ventricular Ejection Fraction Improvement

Earlier studies suggested an improvement in left ventricular ejection fraction (LVEF) following CTO revascularization, as determined by left ventriculography.[20] More contemporary studies have consistently shown improvements in segmental wall function and left ventricular volumes.[21,22] Improvement in overall ejection fraction continues over a period of years, as long as vessel patency is maintained.[22] These studies have generally focused on patients with near normal left ventricular function and have not included patients with histories of large infarctions or significant baseline left ventricular dysfunction.

Survival

Studies have shown that the presence of a CTO has important negative prognostic implications for patient survival, when compared with patients with single or multivessel disease. In numerous observational studies, patients with successful CTO recanalization have demonstrated consistent superiority in survival when compared with patients who have failed revascularization.[23] Unfortunately, there are no randomized trials comparing CTO intervention with medical therapy. Thus, the idea of CTO revascularization providing a survival benefit is still a hypothetical conclusion that is not uniformly accepted by the cardiology community. Still, there are compelling data arguing against CTO as a benign lesion. One study suggests that for patients presenting with stent thrombosis elevation myocardial infarction, the presence of a CTO is poorly tolerated, having a negative impact on 30-day mortality, long-term mortality, and worsening of LVEF.[24]

ALTERNATIVES

The alternatives that should be enumerated for patients considering coronary intervention include medical therapy, coronary artery bypass surgery, and enhanced external counterpulsation. At this point in the conversation, the cardiologist should select his or her recommendation. Consideration should be given to telling the patient the strength of the recommendation and on what basis that recommendation is made: society guidelines, published evidence, patient-specific factors/preferences, physician experience, or another factor.

SUMMARY

The informed consent process for a CTO intervention is similar to the process that is used for other procedures. The elements of the discussion are the same:

- Nature of the procedure
- Risks
- Benefits
- Alternatives.

The conversation should be tailored toward the unique aspects of CTO intervention. These interventions generally last longer than typical coronary interventions, with lower success rates. The expectation should be that procedural success may require multiple procedures. When disclosing risks of the procedure, one should focus on the complications with the greatest severity and those that occur with greatest frequency. An important concept of risk disclosure is the avoidance of being overly general or specific. Excessively broad disclosure may not provide enough information for patients to make an informed choice; being too specific, particularly in documentation, could open the interventionalist to liability for complications that are not mentioned. The discussion of benefits should focus primarily on symptom relief. Although observational data would suggest that there may be survival benefit for recanalization of CTOs, this idea is not universally accepted by the medical community. Finally, the alternatives to the patient's management should be presented, and the rationale for the physician's recommendation should be explained. Once all of the patient's questions are answered, written consent should be obtained and placed in the chart.

In addition to meeting ethical and legal obligations, the informed consent process provides an opportunity to build an alliance with the patient. The cardiologist should adapt his or her discussion with patients to touch upon the elements of informed consent, not only to stream-line the process of moving patients from the office to the catheterization laboratory, but also to provide the necessary information to help patients make decisions about their own medical care.

REFERENCES

1. Beauchamp T, Faden R. History of informed consent. In: Reich WT, editor. Encyclopedia of bioethics. 2nd edition. London: Simon and Schuster Macmillan; 1995. p. 1232–8.

2. Katz J. Legal and ethical issues of consent in health care. In: Reich WT, editor. Encyclopedia of bioethics. 2nd edition. London: Simon and Schuster Macmillan; 1995. p. 1256–63.

3. Arnold RM, Lidz CW. Clinical aspects of consent in health care. In: Reich WT, editor. Encyclopedia of bioethics. 2nd edition. London: Simon and Schuster Macmillan; 1995. p. 1250–6.

4. Prasad A, Rihal CS, Lennon RJ, et al. Trends in outcomes after percutaneous coronary intervention for chronic total occlusions: a 25-year experience from the Mayo Clinic. J Am Coll Cardiol 2007; 49(15):1611–8.

5. Morino Y, Kimura T, Hayashi Y, et al. In-hospital outcomes of contemporary percutaneous coronary intervention in patients with chronic total occlusion insights from the J-CTO Registry (Multicenter CTO Registry in Japan). JACC Cardiovasc Interv 2010; 3(2):143–51.

6. Maiello L, Colombo A, Gianrossi R, et al. Coronary angioplasty of chronic occlusions: factors predictive of procedural success. Am Heart J 1992;124(3): 581–4.

7. Thompson CA, Jayne JE, Robb JF, et al. Retrograde techniques and the impact of operator volume on percutaneous intervention for coronary chronic total occlusions an early U.S. experience. JACC Cardiovasc Interv 2009;2(9):834–42.

8. Rahel BM, Laarman GJ, Kelder JC, et al. Three-year clinical outcome after primary stenting of totally occluded native coronary arteries: a randomized comparison of bare-metal stent implantation with sirolimus-eluting stent implantation for the treatment of total coronary occlusions. Am Heart J 2009; 157(1):149–55.

9. Suero JA, Marso SP, Jones PG, et al. Procedural outcomes and long-term survival among patients undergoing percutaneous coronary intervention of a chronic total occlusion in native coronary arteries: a 20-year experience. J Am Coll Cardiol 2001;38(2): 409–14.

10. Einstein AJ. Effects of radiation exposure from cardiac imaging how good are the data? J Am Coll Cardiol 2012;59(6):553–65.

11. Suzuki S, Furui S, Isshiki T, et al. Patients' skin dose during percutaneous coronary intervention for chronic total occlusion. Catheter Cardiovasc Interv 2008;71(2):160–4.

12. Wagner LK, Eifel PJ, Geise RA. Potential biological effects following high X-ray dose interventional procedures. J Vasc Interv Radiol 1994; 5(1):71–84.

13. Mehran R, Aymong ED, Nikolsky E, et al. A simple risk score for prediction of contrast-induced nephropathy after percutaneous coronary intervention: development and initial validation. J Am Coll Cardiol 2004;44(7):1393–9.

14. Gurm HS, Dixon SR, Smith DE, et al. Renal function-based contrast dosing to define safe limits of radiographic contrast media in patients undergoing percutaneous coronary interventions. J Am Coll Cardiol 2011;58(9):907–14.

15. Olivari Z, Rubartelli P, Piscione F, et al. Immediate results and one-year clinical outcome after percutaneous coronary interventions in chronic total occlusions. J Am Coll Cardiol 2003;41(10):1672–8.

16. Safley DM, Koshy S, Grantham JA, et al. Changes in myocardial ischemic burden following percutaneous coronary intervention of chronic total occlusions. Catheter Cardiovasc Interv 2011;78(3): 337–43.

17. Grantham JA, Marso SP, Spertus J, et al. Chronic total occlusion angioplasty in the United States. JACC Cardiovasc Interv 2009;2(6):479–86.

18. Borgia F, Viceconte N, Ali O, et al. Improved cardiac survival, freedom from mace and angina-related quality of life after successful percutaneous recanalization of coronary artery chronic total occlusions. Int J Cardiol 2011. [Epub ahead of print].

19. Mehran R, Claessen BE, Godino C, et al. Long-term outcome of percutaneous coronary intervention for chronic total occlusions. JACC Cardiovasc Interv 2011;4(9):952–61.

20. Chung CM, Nakamura S, Tanaka K, et al. Effect of recanalization of chronic total occlusions on global and regional left ventricular function in patients with or without previous myocardial infarction. Catheter Cardiovasc Interv 2003;60(3):368–74.

21. Baks T, van Geuns RJ, Duncker DJ, et al. Prediction of left ventricular function after drug-eluting stent implantation for chronic total coronary occlusions. J Am Coll Cardiol 2006;47(4):721–5.

22. Kirschbaum SW, Baks T, van den Ent M, et al. Evaluation of left ventricular function three years after percutaneous recanalization of chronic total coronary occlusions. Am J Cardiol 2008;101(2):179–85.

23. Joyal D, Afilalo J, Rinfret S. Effectiveness of recanalization of chronic total occlusions: a systematic review and meta-analysis. Am Heart J 2010;160(1):179–87.

24. Claessen BE, van der Schaaf RJ, Verouden NJ, et al. Evaluation of the effect of a concurrent chronic total occlusion on long-term mortality and left ventricular function in patients after primary percutaneous coronary intervention. JACC Cardiovasc Interv 2009; 2(11):1128–34.

Complications of Chronic Total Occlusion Angioplasty

Emmanouil S. Brilakis, MD, PhD[a],*,
Dimitri Karmpaliotis, MD[b], Vishal Patel, MD[a],
Subhash Banerjee, MD[a]

KEYWORDS

- Percutaneous coronary intervention • Chronic total occlusion • Stents • Complications

KEY POINTS

- Acute chronic total occlusion (CTO) intervention complications can be coronary artery–related (such as coronary occlusion, coronary perforation, or equipment loss or entrapment), cardiac noncoronary (such as periprocedural myocardial infarction, arrhythmias, and tamponade), or noncardiac (such as vascular access complications, systemic embolization contrast-induced nephropathy and allergic reactions, and radiation-induced injury).
- There are 3 main perforation types: (1) main vessel perforation (which may require implantation of a covered stent), (2) distal wire perforation, and (3) collateral vessel perforation (which may require coil embolization).
- Long-term, CTO interventions can be complicated by in-stent restenosis, stent thrombosis, or coronary aneurysm formation.
- CTO interventions may require significant radiation exposure to the patient; therefore, careful follow-up should be performed to diagnose radiation-induced skin injury in patients who receive >5 Gy air kerma.

Percutaneous coronary intervention (PCI) has revolutionized the treatment of coronary artery disease, but as any other medical procedure, PCI carries a risk for complications. This is also true for chronic total occlusion (CTO) PCI. Such complications can be classified according to timing (as acute and long term) and according to location (cardiac coronary, cardiac noncoronary, and noncardiac) (**Figs. 1–3** and **Table 1**).[1–5] In the present study, we review the possible complications of CTO PCI and present prevention and treatment strategies.

ACUTE COMPLICATIONS
Acute Coronary Complications

Acute vessel closure
Donor vessel closure during retrograde CTO PCI Although by definition CTO signifies that the target vessel is occluded, CTO PCI can be complicated by occlusion of a nontarget vessel, for example during retrograde CTO PCI (**Fig. 4**). Because the nontarget vessel may supply the entire coronary perfusion (especially in patients who have not had coronary artery bypass graft

Conflict of interest disclosures related to this manuscript: Dr Brilakis: Speaker honoraria from St Jude Medical and Terumo; research support from Abbott Vascular; salary from Medtronic (spouse). Dr Karmpaliotis: speaker honoraria from Abbott Vascular; his institution (Piedmont Heart Institute) has received educational grant from Bridgepoint Medical. Dr Patel: None. Dr Banerjee: Speaker honoraria from St Jude Medical, Medtronic, and Johnson & Johnson and research support from Boston Scientific and The Medicines Company.
a Division of Cardiology, VA North Texas Health Care System, The University of Texas Southwestern Medical Center at Dallas, 4500 South Lancaster Road, Dallas, TX 75216, USA; b Piedmont Heart Institute, 275 Collier Road North West, Suite 300, Atlanta, GA 30309, USA
* Corresponding author.
E-mail address: esbrilakis@yahoo.com

Intervent Cardiol Clin 1 (2012) 373–389
doi:10.1016/j.iccl.2012.04.006
2211-7458/12/$ – see front matter Published by Elsevier Inc.

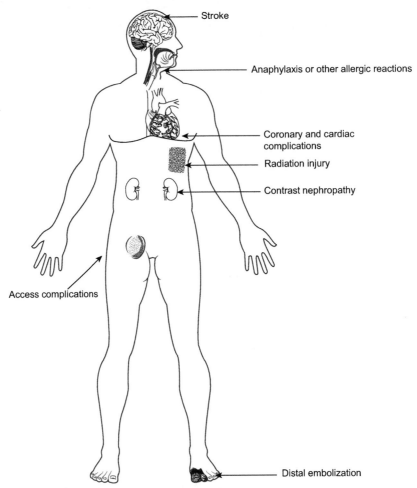

Fig. 1. Complications of chronic total occlusion interventions.

surgery), its occlusion can cause severe ischemia leading to acute hemodynamic decompensation, urgent coronary artery bypass graft surgery (see **Fig. 4**), or death.[6] Donor vessel occlusion can be caused by guide catheter–induced injury, especially during equipment withdrawal that causes the guide to deeply engage the vessel. Moreover, donor vessel thrombosis can occur during long procedures requiring coronary artery intubation by microcatheters or guide wires. Donor vessel injury can be prevented by

- Careful attention to the position of the guide catheter (especially during equipment manipulations) and to the pressure waveform (to prevent pressure dampening)
- Not using guide catheters with side holes to engage the CTO donor vessel, as they may mask suboptimal guide catheter position
- Maintaining high activated clotting time (the authors use >350 seconds during retrograde CTO PCI)

- Avoiding the retrograde approach through diffusely diseased donor vessels
- Back-bleeding the guide catheter once balloon-trapping techniques are used to minimize the risk for air embolization.

Although the left internal mammary artery (LIMA) is seldom used for retrograde CTO PCI, its wiring may be complicated by acute closure, when the LIMA tortuosity is straightened by use of the coronary guide wire.[7] Tortuous LIMA grafts should not be used for retrograde CTO PCI to minimize the risk for LIMA injury or ischemia owing to decreased antegrade flow.

Aortic dissection Aortic dissection can complicate any PCI, but is more common with CTO PCI and mostly occurs in the right coronary artery (**Fig. 5**).[8] It is usually a result of guide catheter trauma (especially when large-caliber guide catheters with aggressive shapes, such as Amplatz, are used), but may also be caused by forceful contrast

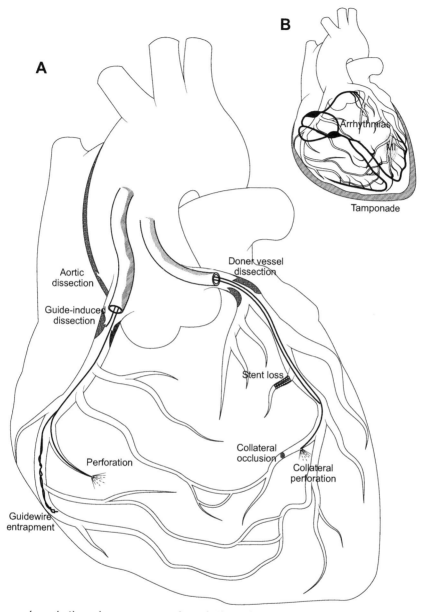

Fig. 2. Coronary (*panel A*) and noncoronary (*panel B*) cardiac complications of chronic total occlusion interventions.

injection through a wedged catheter, or by balloon rupture. Use of guide catheters with side holes and/or careful attention to avoid injecting when guide catheter pressure is dampened may help prevent this complication.

If aortic dissection occurs, it is important to (1) stop further coronary injections (as they can expand the dissection plane) and (2) rapidly stent the ostium of the coronary artery to "seal" the dissection. In cases with difficult visualization or placement of an ostial stent, intravascular ultrasonography can assist localizing the dissection port of entry and

ensuring adequate ostial coverage.[9] Subsequently, (3) the dissection should be carefully followed by noninvasive imaging (such as computed tomography or transesophageal echocardiography) to ensure that it has stabilized. Emergency surgery is rarely needed except in patients who develop aortic regurgitation, tamponade owing to rupture into the pericardium, or extension of the dissection.[8]

Side branch occlusion Side branch occlusion can occur during CTO PCI, especially when subintimal dissection/reentry strategies are used, and is

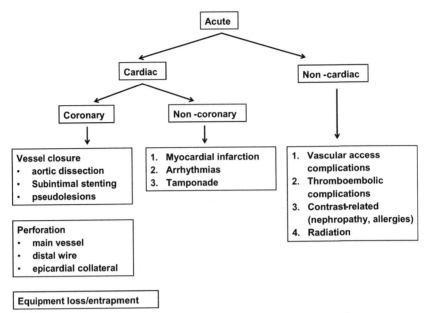

Fig. 3. Classification of complications of coronary chronic total occlusion interventions.

associated with higher frequency of post-PCI myocardial infarction.[8] That is why if a dissection/reentry strategy is used, it is important to minimize the extent of the subintimal dissection by reentering into the true lumen at the most proximal location possible: this strategy has been named Limited Antegrade Subintimal Tracking and redirection (LAST).[10] Moreover, using the CrossBoss catheter (Bridgepoint Medical, Minneapolis, MN) may minimize the extent of subintimal dissection and facilitate reentry attempts. The presence of a coronary bifurcation at the distal CTO cap may favor use of a primary retrograde approach to minimize the risk for side branch occlusion during antegrade crossing attempts.

Occlusion of a single, large collateral (usually epicardial) may cause severe ischemia and hemodynamic instability; therefore, there should be a high threshold for performing retrograde CTO PCI through such collaterals. Moreover, successful CTO recanalization results in rapid "de-recruitment" of the collateral circulation, resulting in severe ischemia, if the vessel reoccludes.[11]

Distal vessel dissection Distal vessel injury can occur when subintimal wire crossing causes

Table 1
Frequency of complications among the largest reported series of CTO interventions

Author	Year	N (Patients/ Lesions)	Success %	Retrograde %	Tamponade %	MI %	Emergent CABG %	Radiation Dermatitis %
Suero et al[1] (MAHI)	2001	2007/NR	69.9	0	0.5	2.4	0.7	NR
Prasad et al[2] (Mayo Clinic)	2007	1262/NR[a]	70	0	0.8	5	0.7	NR
Rathore et al[3] (Toyohashi)	2009	806/902	87.5	17.1	1.5	3.0	0.2	NR
Morino et al[4] (J-CTO)	2010	498/528	87.7	25.7	0.4	2.3	0	0
Galassi et al[5] (ERCTO)	2011	1914/1983	82.9	11.8	0.5	1.3	0.1	NR

Abbreviations: CABG, coronary artery bypass graft; CTO, chronic total occlusion; ERCTO, European CTO Club; J-CTO, Japan CTO Club; MAHI, Mid America Heart Institute; NR, not reported.
  [a] Outcomes from 152 patients from the drug-eluting stent era are presented.

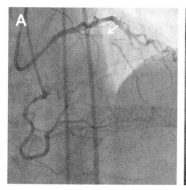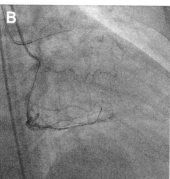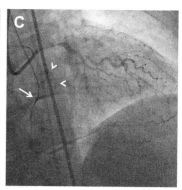

Fig. 4. Donor vessel injury during retrograde chronic total occlusion intervention. Coronary angiography using dual injection demonstrating a chronic total occlusion of the mid left anterior descending artery (*A, arrow*). After antegrade crossing attempts failed, retrograde crossing was attempted through the right coronary artery (*B*). Proximal right coronary artery dissection occurred (*C, arrow*) extending into the aorta (*C, arrowheads*) necessitating emergency coronary artery bypass graft surgery.

subintimal hematoma that compresses the true lumen. If reentry fails, it may be best to wait for 2 to 3 months before reattempting CTO PCI, to allow time for healing of the dissection.

Perforation

Coronary perforation is one of the most feared complications of CTO PCI, as it can lead to pericardial effusion causing tamponade, often necessitating emergency pericardiocentesis and,

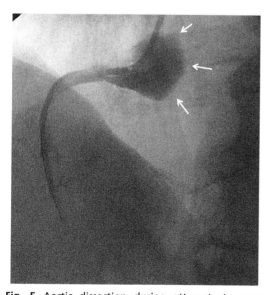

Fig. 5. Aortic dissection during attempts to cross a right coronary artery chronic total occlusion (*arrows*). The procedure was stopped and the patient had an uneventful recovery. Transesophageal echocardiography the following day demonstrated resolution of the dissection.

rarely, cardiac surgery to be controlled. Although coronary perforations are common in CTO PCI (27.6% in one series[3]), most perforations do not have serious consequences, and the risk of tamponade is low, approximately 0.5% (see **Table 1**).

Coronary perforations have traditionally been classified according to severity using the Ellis classification,[12] as follows:

- Class 1: a crater extending outside the lumen only in the absence of linear staining angiographically suggestive of dissection
- Class 2: Pericardial or myocardial blush without a 1 mm or larger exit hole
- Class 3: Frank streaming of contrast through a 1 mm or larger exit hole
- Class 3-cavity spilling: Perforation into an anatomic cavity chamber, such as the coronary sinus, the right ventricle, and so forth

Coronary perforations may additionally be classified according to location, which has important implications regarding management. There are 3 main perforation locations: (1) main vessel perforation, (2) distal wire perforation, and (3) collateral vessel perforation, in either a septal or epicardial collateral (**Fig. 6**).

Main vessel perforation Main vessel perforation can be caused by implantation of oversized stents or by high-pressure balloon inflations. Another mechanism is wire exit from the vessel followed by inadvertent advancement of equipment (such as balloons or microcatheters) into the pericardial space. Whereas wire perforation alone seldom causes blood extravasation and pericardial effusion (because it creates a very small, self-sealing hole) catheter/balloon advancement over the wire enlarges the hole,

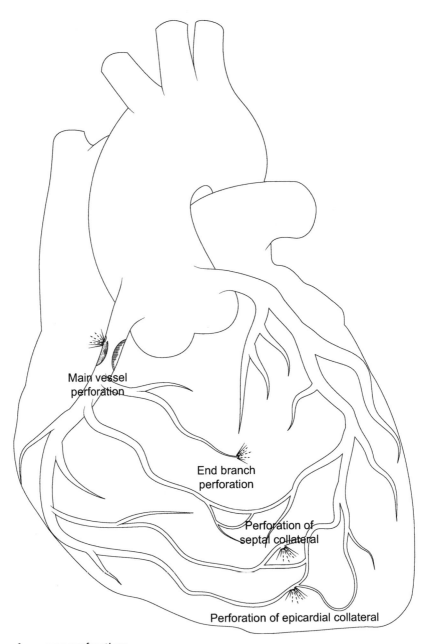

Fig. 6. Types of coronary perforations.

increasing the risk for blood extravasation. Occasionally the contrast extravasation may not occur until after a stent is placed over the perforated area.

As with any perforation, if a main vessel perforation occurs, the first step is to inflate a balloon proximal to the perforation to stop the bleeding (**Figs. 7** and **8**). If extravasation persists in spite of anticoagulation reversal and prolonged balloon inflations, then a covered stent may need to be deployed.[13] The only stent that is currently approved for use in the United States is the Jostent Graftmaster covered stent (Abbott Vascular, Santa Clara, CA, USA which is approved through a humanitarian device exemption).[14] Operators should be aware of the following about this stent:

- It is bulky and difficult to deliver, requiring at least a 7-French guide catheter and excellent guide catheter support

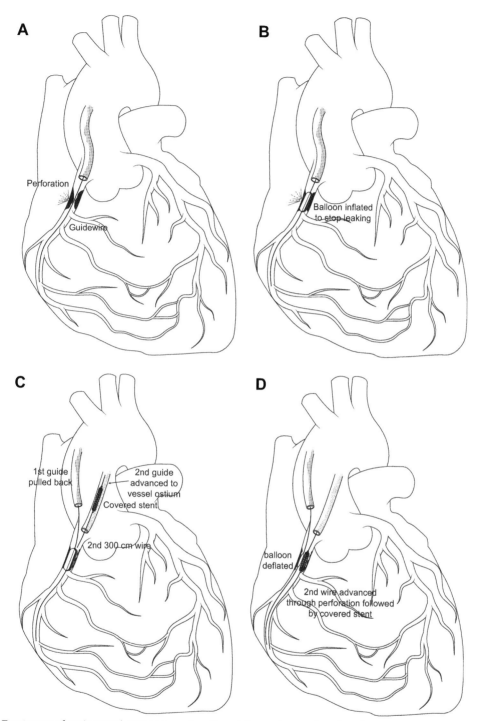

Fig. 7. Treatment of main vessel coronary perforation. After main vessel perforation occurs (*A*), a balloon is inflated at the perforation site to stop bleeding into the pericardium (*B*). A second guide catheter is advanced to the coronary artery ostium with a covered stent over a 300-cm guide wire (*C*). The first guide is withdrawn and the balloon deflated followed by wiring of the coronary artery with the second guide wire and advancement of the covered stent to the perforation site (*D*). Deployment of the covered stent (*E*) results in sealing of the perforation (*F*).

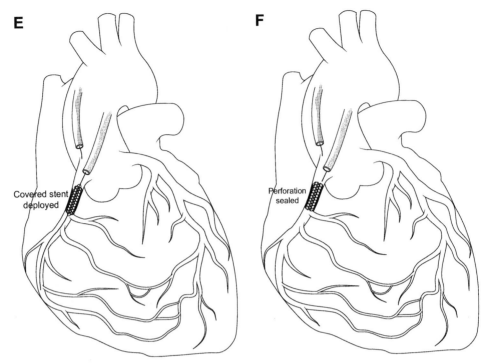

Fig. 7. (*continued*)

- It is available in diameters of 3 to 5 mm and lengths between 9 and 26 mm
- It is available only as an over-the-wire system (ie, it requires a 300-cm-long wire for delivery)
- It may be difficult to advance it through previously deployed stents, necessitating techniques such as distal anchor and use of delivery catheters, such as the Guideliner catheter (Vascular Solutions, Minneapolis, MN) (ideally the larger 8-French Guideliner)
- It frequently requires use of a dual-catheter technique to minimize bleeding into the

pericardium while preparing for covered stent delivery and deployment (see **Fig. 7**).[15] In this technique, a balloon is inserted through one guide catheter and inflated proximal to the perforation, preventing bleeding, while a second guide catheter with the covered stent is advanced through the aorta to engage the same coronary ostium, next to the previous guiding catheter. The covered stent is advanced on a new wire through that second guiding catheter and placed just proximally to the sealing balloon, which is briefly deflated

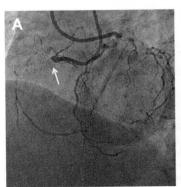
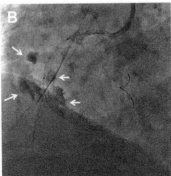
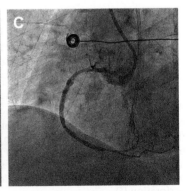

Fig. 8. Example of main vessel perforation. A right coronary artery chronic total occlusion (*A, arrows*) was successfully crossed antegradely. Poststenting angiography demonstrated a main vessel perforation with active bleeding into the pericardium (*B, arrows*). Emergency pericardiocentesis was performed and after implantation of a covered stent, the bleeding stopped (*C*).

and withdrawn proximally to allow passage of the wire and the covered stent. Use of this dual-guide catheter technique minimizes the time that the perforation remains unsealed.[15]

Distal wire perforation Distal wire perforations (**Figs. 9** and **10**) are caused by inadvertent advancement of a guide wire into a distal small branch. Stiff, tapered, and polymer-jacketed guide wires are more likely to cause such perforations. Distal wire perforation can be prevented by

- Meticulous attention to the distal wire position (which may be challenging when collimation is used to reduce radiation dose) and
- Rapid exchange of stiff or polymer-jacketed guide wires for soft workhorse wires early after CTO crossing.

If distal wire perforation is not sealed by prolonged balloon inflation and by reversing anticoagulation, embolization of the bleeding vessel may be required, using coils,[16] subcutaneous fat, thrombus,[17] or other materials (see **Fig. 9**). Alternatively, a microcatheter may be advanced to the perforation site and suction applied, collapsing the vessel to achieve hemostasis.[18]

Patients with distal wire perforation should be monitored closely and should not receive a glycoprotein IIb/IIIa inhibitor, as tamponade may not develop until hours after the end of PCI.

Collateral vessel perforation Perforation of an epicardial collateral branch is a serious complication of retrograde CTO PCI, as it can rapidly lead to tamponade and may be particularly difficult to control. In contrast, perforation of septal collaterals is unlikely to have adverse consequences,[6] although septal hematomas[19] and even tamponade[17] have been reported following septal wire perforation. Septal rupture/hematoma has been reported to occur in up to 6.9% of cases in a single series of patients treated with a retrograde approach.[20] In case reports, septal hematomas have caused asymptomatic bigeminy and severe chest pain, appear as an echo-free space in the interventricular septum on transthoracic echocardiography, and resolve spontaneously.[21] Careful attention should be paid to the collateral branch course, as a collateral that appears to be septal may in reality be epicardial. Moreover, perforation into the coronary sinus has been reported during attempts to cross a septal collateral.[22] Perforation into a cardiac chamber usually does not cause complications; however, balloon dilation or advancement of additional equipment should be avoided.

Wiring epicardial collaterals should be performed only by operators experienced in the retrograde approach. Epicardial collateral wiring is safer in patients with prior coronary bypass graft surgery or other surgery that required pericardial entry, as bleeding may be contained within pericardial "pockets."

In contrast to septal collaterals, epicardial collaterals should never be dilated to minimize the risk of perforation; however, the septal dilator catheter (Corsair, Asahi Intecc, Aichi, Japan) can be used in epicardial collaterals, paying careful attention to avoid catheter advancement in front of the guide wire. If an epicardial collateral is ruptured or perforated and bleeding cannot be stopped by reversing anticoagulation, the bleeding collateral may need to be embolized. Embolization should be performed on both sides of the perforation, as blood flow can continue retrogradely in spite of occluding the antegrade collateral limb (**Fig. 11**). This may not be feasible in cases in which the CTO cannot and has not been recanalized (**Fig. 12**), occasionally necessitating surgery if bleeding does not cease with conservative treatment.

Prevention of perforations Prevention and minimization of the risk of bleeding through a perforation are critical, as perforations may often be small and unrecognized during the procedure, but manifest as tamponade hours or even days afterward. This can be accomplished in several ways:

- Using unfractionated heparin for anticoagulation, as it can be reversed in case of perforation, in contrast to bivalirudin
- Not administering glycoprotein IIb/IIIa inhibitors during CTO PCI, even after successful crossing and stenting, as they may cause an unrecognized perforation to bleed. Although large perforations are self-evident on angiography, small perforations (especially distal wire perforations) may be difficult to detect, especially when collimation is used to minimize radiation exposure.
- Paying careful attention to distal wire position during attempts to deliver equipment, especially when stiff and polymer wires are used, as those are more likely to perforate compared with workhorse guide wires. Using the trapping technique can minimize wire movement during equipment exchanges.
- Exchanging a stiff or polymer-jacketed guide wire for a workhorse wire immediately after confirmation of successful crossing.

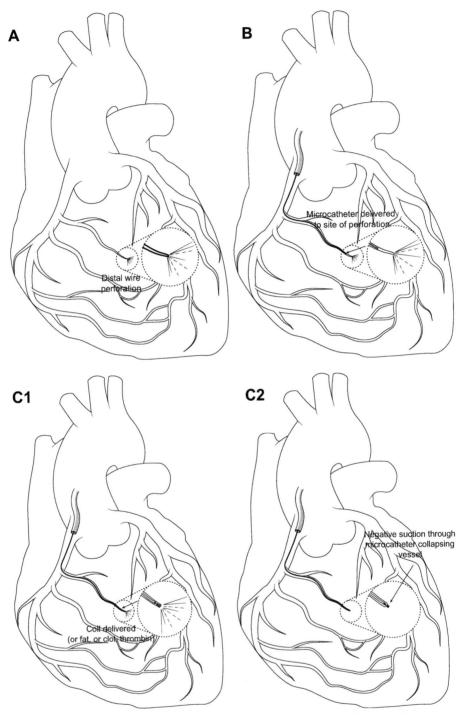

Fig. 9. Management of distal wire perforation. To treat a distal guide wire perforation (*A*), a microcatheter is advanced proximal to the perforation (*B*) and either a coil (of other material, such as subcutaneous fat) is released (*C1*) or suction is applied through the microcatheter, collapsing the vessel (*C2*), and sealing the perforation.

General treatment of perforations Location-specific treatments have been described previously according to the type of perforation (main vessel, distal wire, and collateral vessel perforation). General measures that can decrease the risk of continued bleeding into the pericardium include the following:

- Reversal of anticoagulation by administering protamine (in patients who have not received

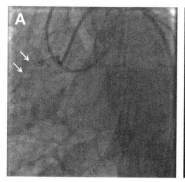 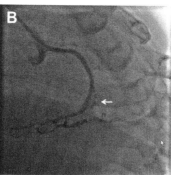 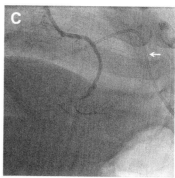

Fig. 10. Example of distal wire perforation. A right coronary artery chronic total occlusion (*A, arrows*) was successfully crossed antegradely using a 12 g stiff guide wire. Poststenting angiography demonstrated a side branch perforation with active bleeding into the pericardium (*B, arrows*). Emergency pericardiocentesis was performed (*C, arrow*). Delivery of a covered stent failed, but after prolonged balloon inflation and reversal of anticoagulation, the side branch bleeding stopped.

neutral protamine Hagedorn insulin in the past). Platelet administration can help reverse the effect of abciximab, but glycoprotein IIb/IIIa inhibitors should not be administered during CTO PCI.

- Administration of intravenous fluids and pressors, and possibly atropine if the patient develops bradycardia caused by a vagal reaction.
- Appropriate timing for performing pericardiocentesis. Hemodynamic instability requires immediate pericardiocentesis, yet smaller size pericardial effusions may be best managed conservatively, as the elevated pericardial pressure, owing to the entrance of blood into the pericardial space, may help "tamponade the perforation site" and minimize the risk for further bleeding.
- Pericardiocentesis can frequently be performed using radiographic guidance because of contrast exit into the pericardial space. Echocardiography remains important for assessing the size of pericardial effusion and the result of pericardiocentesis, and for determining whether pericardial bleeding continues. Use of echocardiographic contrast agents can be useful for detecting ongoing bleeding into the pericardial space
- Cardiac surgery notification. If pericardial bleeding continues in spite of percutaneous management attempts, cardiac surgery may be required to identify and control the site of bleeding.

Equipment loss or entrapment

Equipment delivery may be challenging in CTO vessels that are frequently tortuous and calcified. Stent loss or wire entrapment may ensue. The risk

for stent loss[23] or wire entrapment[24] may be particularly increased when retrograde wiring and stent delivery is attempted. As with non-CTO PCI, familiarity with various techniques and equipment related to stent retrieval, such as using various snares, is important for successful management.[25] Often "crushing" or deployment of the lost stent or encasing of the guide wire fragment with stents[24] may be preferable to retrieval. Intravascular imaging is important to ensure that there is adequate coverage of the lost equipment and that there is no wire unraveling extending proximally in the coronary artery or even into the aorta.

Acute Cardiac Noncoronary Complications

Noncoronary cardiac complications include periprocedural myocardial infarction, arrhythmias, and tamponade. Tamponade is the result of coronary perforation and has been discussed in detail previously. Arrhythmias can complicate CTO PCI, but are infrequent and are usually caused by ischemia.

Postprocedural myocardial infarction is an infrequent complication of CTO PCI (see **Table 1**); however, its incidence may be underdiagnosed because of the lack of systematic screening. Several mechanisms may lead to periprocedural myocardial infarction during CTO PCI:

- Side branch occlusion at or proximal to the CTO[26]
- Collateral vessel occlusion or injury, especially when collateral flow is provided by a single collateral (usually epicardial)
- Injury of the target vessel distal to the CTO caused by subintimal wire passage; this may be worsened if subintimal stenting is inadvertently performed

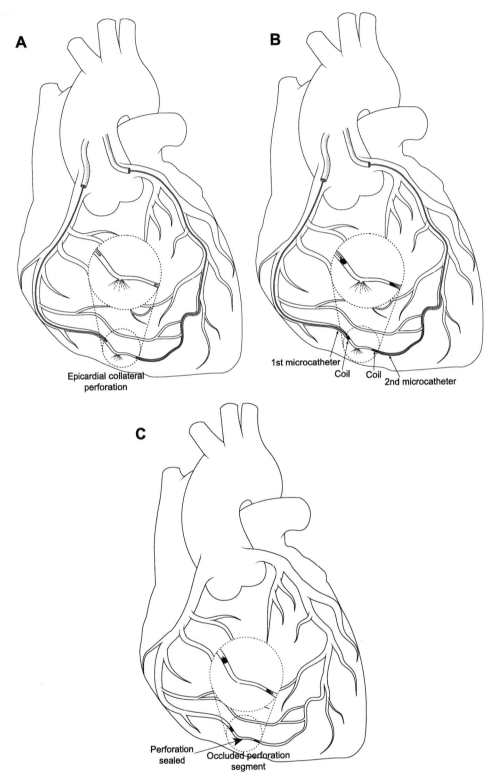

Fig. 11. Management of epicardial collateral perforation. To treat an epicardial collateral perforation (*A*), 2 microcatheters are advanced through both the antegrade and retrograde guide catheter on both ends of the perforation site and a coil is released via both microcatheters (*B*), sealing the perforation (*C*).

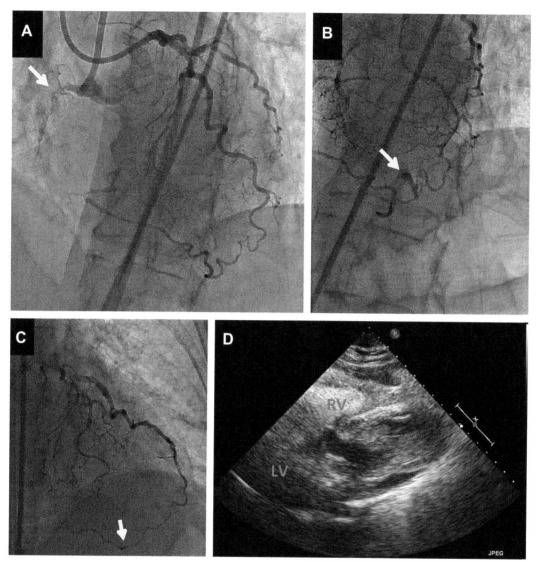

Fig. 12. Example of epicardial collateral perforation. A retrograde crossing attempt was performed to treat a patient with a proximal right coronary artery chronic total occlusion (*A, arrow*); however, during attempts to cross the epicardial collateral from the diagonal to the right posterior descending artery, perforation occurred (*B, arrow*). After prolonged balloon inflation and reversal of anticoagulation, bleeding through the perforation stopped (*C, arrow*), as confirmed by injection of echocardiographic contrast (*D*).

- Donor vessel injury and/or thrombus and air embolization, as discussed earlier in the section "Donor vessel closure during retrograde CTO PCI."

Compared with antegrade, retrograde CTO PCI may be associated with higher rates of postprocedural cardiac biomarker elevation, but it is unclear whether this has an impact on acute and long-term clinical outcomes. Meticulous attention to prevent vessel occlusion and perforation and equipment loss can help minimize the risk for post-PCI myocardial infarction.

Other Acute General Complications

CTO interventions are subject to the same risks as non-CTO interventions.

Vascular access complications can occur, especially given the frequent use of large sheaths in both femoral arteries. The risk of such complications could be reduced by using radial access, usually as the second arterial access for dual injection, although some operators routinely perform biradial CTO interventions.[27] However, femoral access can provide more support for retrograde collateral channel crossing and retrograde CTO

PCI. Using fluoroscopy or ultrasonography to choose the femoral arterial puncture site can also be useful. Routine performance of iliofemoral angiography at the time of diagnostic angiography before referral for CTO PCI may be useful for optimal selection of the vascular access sites.

Systemic thromboembolic complications can complicate any cardiac catheterization, including CTO PCI. Careful attention to aspiration of the guide catheters after advancement through the aorta and use of 0.065 guide wires for guide advancement may help minimize "scraping" of the aorta and peripheral embolization. Moreover, careful attention to anticoagulation (which is especially important for retrograde CTO PCI to minimize the risk of donor vessel thrombosis) can minimize the risk of catheter thrombus formation and subsequent embolization.

Contrast allergic reactions can often be prevented by using a premedication regimen. Such a regimen usually includes a steroid, an H1 antihistamine blocker, such as diphenhydramine, and an H2 antihistamine blocker, such as cimetidine. Limiting the volume of contrast administered and routine fluid administration before CTO PCI can help minimize the risk for contrast nephropathy.

Finally, radiation injury is of particular importance to CTO PCI, which often requires extensive fluoroscopy use. There is increased awareness and recognition of radiation-related injury, both acute (mainly skin injury) or delayed (increased risk for cancer and cataracts) for both the patient and the operator.[28] Radiation skin injury is a deterministic effect (ie, it will happen if a certain radiation threshold is exceeded), whereas the risk of cancer is stochastic (ie, there is increased lifetime risk for this occurring). Although commonly used, fluoroscopy time is not a good measure of radiation exposure, because the actual administered radiation dose depends on multiple factors, such as the weight of the patient, the use of collimation, the imaging angles used, and the use of cineangiography. The best radiation measure for radiation exposure as it relates to the risk of skin injury is air kerma dose. There is significant risk for skin injury if more than 5-Gy air kerma dose is administered, which is virtually certain if more than 15 Gy is administered.[28] That is why radiation exposure should be carefully monitored by the operator throughout the procedure and the procedure may need to be terminated if a prespecified threshold (approximately 7–10 Gy) is reached.

Several measures can be taken to minimize radiation exposure during CTO PCI[29]:

1. Limit fluoroscopy use (for example, by using the "trapping technique for equipment exchanges)

2. Limit use of cine-angiography by using the image store function, which is available in most modern x-ray equipment
3. Use of low magnification
4. Use of collimation
5. Use of 7.5 frames per second fluoroscopy
6. Frequent rotation of the image intensifier to minimize the exposure of each area of the skin
7. Optimize the position of the table (as high as possible) and the image intensifier (as close to the patient as possible)
8. Avoidance of steep angles
9. Injecting the CTO collateral donor vessel before starting cine-angiography
10. Use of radiation monitors that provide real-time feedback on operator radiation exposure
11. Use additional shielding, such as the X-drape (AADCO Medical, Randolph, VT)
12. Pay continuous attention to the air kerma radiation dose and use it to modify the procedural plan.

Patients who are exposed to more than 5 Gy of air kerma dose radiation should be carefully followed-up to detect a possibly skin injury. Air kerma dose of more than 15 Gy is considered a sentinel event by the Joint Commission for Hospital Accreditation.

LONG-TERM COMPLICATIONS

Similar to non-CTO interventions, patients who undergo CTO PCI may subsequently experience in-stent restenosis or stent thrombosis. The CTO lesion in-stent restenosis rates were very high when bare-metal stents were used, resulting in repeat revascularization rates of 19% to 53%.[30] Use of drug-eluting stents significantly reduced the restenosis risk; however, the need for repeat target vessel revascularization remained significant (3%–18%), likely in part because of long stent length and in part because of stent undersizing, as the target vessel is frequently underexpanded owing to chronic hypoperfusion. Although the risk of stent thrombosis could also be expected to be higher in CTO lesions, the rate was similar between bare-metal and drug-eluting–treated lesions.[30] Many operators routinely administer more than 12 months of dual antiplatelet therapy in patients who undergo successful CTO PCI, although the safety and efficacy of the regimen in this high-risk patient group remains unknown.

Late coronary artery aneurysm formation may complicate CTO PCI, possibly with higher frequency in patients who undergo subintimal CTO crossing (**Fig. 13**). Coronary artery aneurysms were seen in 7.3% of patients in whom retrograde intervention was performed versus

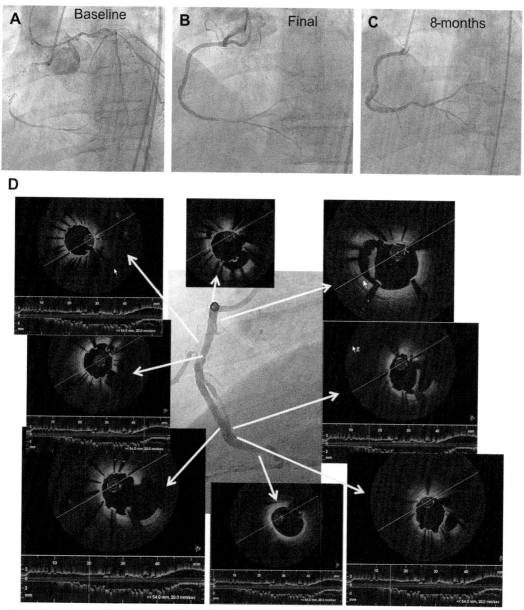

Fig. 13. Late coronary artery aneurysm formation after chronic total occlusion intervention (*A*). A right coronary artery chronic total occlusion was successfully crossed using a dissection/reentry strategy and stented using 3 drug-eluting stents (*B*). Repeat angiography performed 8 months later revealed a mid right coronary artery aneurysm (*C*), as confirmed by optical coherence tomography (*D*). The patient remained asymptomatic and repeat coronary angiography and long-term dual antiplatelet therapy was recommended.

2.6% of patients in whom antegrade intervention was performed among 560 patients undergoing CTO PCI in Japan.[31] Treatment of such aneurysms is controversial because of lack of natural history data. At present, a reasonable approach is to continue dual antiplatelet therapy and perform serial angiographic and intravascular imaging (with intravascular ultrasonography or ideally with optical coherence tomography that has higher resolution), with aneurysm sealing limited to patients with large aneurysms or aneurysms that enlarge during follow-up.[32]

REFERENCES

1. Suero JA, Marso SP, Jones PG, et al. Procedural outcomes and long-term survival among patients undergoing percutaneous coronary intervention of

a chronic total occlusion in native coronary arteries: a 20-year experience. J Am Coll Cardiol 2001;38: 409–14.

2. Prasad A, Rihal CS, Lennon RJ, et al. Trends in outcomes after percutaneous coronary intervention for chronic total occlusions: a 25-year experience from the Mayo Clinic. J Am Coll Cardiol 2007;49:1611–8.

3. Rathore S, Matsuo H, Terashima M, et al. Procedural and in-hospital outcomes after percutaneous coronary intervention for chronic total occlusions of coronary arteries 2002 to 2008: impact of novel guidewire techniques. JACC Cardiovasc Interv 2009;2:489–97.

4. Morino Y, Kimura T, Hayashi Y, et al. In-hospital outcomes of contemporary percutaneous coronary intervention in patients with chronic total occlusion insights from the J-CTO Registry (Multicenter CTO Registry in Japan). JACC Cardiovasc Interv 2010; 3:143–51.

5. Galassi AR, Tomasello SD, Reifart N, et al. In-hospital outcomes of percutaneous coronary intervention in patients with chronic total occlusion: insights from the ERCTO (European Registry of Chronic Total Occlusion) registry. EuroIntervention 2011;7:472–9.

6. Lee NH, Seo HS, Choi JH, et al. Recanalization strategy of retrograde angioplasty in patients with coronary chronic total occlusion. Analysis of 24 cases, focusing on technical aspects and complications. Int J Cardiol 2010;144(2):219–29.

7. Lichtenwalter C, Banerjee S, Brilakis ES. Dual guide catheter technique for treating native coronary artery lesions through tortuous internal mammary grafts: separating equipment delivery from target lesion visualization. J Invasive Cardiol 2010;22: E78–81.

8. Carstensen S, Ward MR. Iatrogenic aortocoronary dissection: the case for immediate aortoostial stenting. Heart Lung Circ 2008;17:325–9.

9. Abdou SM, Wu CJ. Treatment of aortocoronary dissection complicating anomalous origin right coronary artery and chronic total intervention with intravascular ultrasound guided stenting. Catheter Cardiovasc Interv 2011;78(6):914–9.

10. Lombardi WL. Retrograde PCI: what will they think of next? J Invasive Cardiol 2009;21:543.

11. Zimarino M, Ausiello A, Contegiacomo G, et al. Rapid decline of collateral circulation increases susceptibility to myocardial ischemia: the trade-off of successful percutaneous recanalization of chronic total occlusions. J Am Coll Cardiol 2006;48:59–65.

12. Ellis SG, Ajluni S, Arnold AZ, et al. Increased coronary perforation in the new device era. Incidence, classification, management, and outcome. Circulation 1994;90:2725–30.

13. Briguori C, Nishida T, Anzuini A, et al. Emergency polytetrafluoroethylene-covered stent implantation to treat coronary ruptures. Circulation 2000;102: 3028–31.

14. Romaguera R, Waksman R. Covered stents for coronary perforations: is there enough evidence? Catheter Cardiovasc Interv 2011;78:246–53.

15. Ben-Gal Y, Weisz G, Collins MB, et al. Dual catheter technique for the treatment of severe coronary artery perforations. Catheter Cardiovasc Interv 2010;75: 708–12.

16. Rathore S, Katoh O, Matsuo H, et al. Retrograde percutaneous recanalization of chronic total occlusion of the coronary arteries: procedural outcomes and predictors of success in contemporary practice. Circ Cardiovasc Interv 2009;2:124–32.

17. Matsumi J, Adachi K, Saito S. A unique complication of the retrograde approach in angioplasty for chronic total occlusion of the coronary artery. Catheter Cardiovasc Interv 2008;72:371–8.

18. Yasuoka Y, Sasaki T. Successful collapse vessel treatment with a syringe for thrombus-aspiration after the guidewire-induced coronary artery perforation. Cardiovasc Revasc Med 2010;11(263):e1–3.

19. Lin TH, Wu DK, Su HM, et al. Septum hematoma: a complication of retrograde wiring in chronic total occlusion. Int J Cardiol 2006;113:e64–6.

20. Sianos G, Barlis P, Di Mario C, et al. European experience with the retrograde approach for the recanalisation of coronary artery chronic total occlusions. A report on behalf of the euroCTO club. EuroIntervention 2008;4:84–92.

21. Fairley SL, Donnelly PM, Hanratty CG, et al. Images in cardiovascular medicine. Interventricular septal hematoma and ventricular septal defect after retrograde intervention for a chronic total occlusion of a left anterior descending coronary artery. Circulation 2010;122:e518–21.

22. Sachdeva R, Hughes B, Uretsky BF. Retrograde approach to a totally occluded right coronary artery via a septal perforator artery: the tale of a long and winding wire. J Invasive Cardiol 2010;22:E65–6.

23. Utsunomiya M, Kobayashi T, Nakamura S. Case of dislodged stent lost in septal channel during stent delivery in complex chronic total occlusion of right coronary artery. J Invasive Cardiol 2009;21: E229–33.

24. Sianos G, Papafaklis MI. Septal wire entrapment during recanalisation of a chronic total occlusion with the retrograde approach. Hellenic J Cardiol 2011;52:79–83.

25. Brilakis ES, Best PJ, Elesber AA, et al. Incidence, retrieval methods, and outcomes of stent loss during percutaneous coronary intervention: a large single-center experience. Catheter Cardiovasc Interv 2005;66:333–40.

26. Paizis I, Manginas A, Voudris V, et al. Percutaneous coronary intervention for chronic total occlusions: the

role of side-branch obstruction. EuroIntervention 2009; 4:600–6.

27. Rinfret S, Joyal D, Nguyen C, et al. Retrograde recanalization of chronic total occlusions from the transradial approach; early Canadian experience. Cathet Cardiovasc Interv 2011;78:366–74.

28. Chambers CE, Fetterly KA, Holzer R, et al. Radiation safety program for the cardiac catheterization laboratory. Catheter Cardiovasc Interv 2011;77:546–56.

29. Chambers CE. Radiation dose in percutaneous coronary intervention OUCH did that hurt? JACC Cardiovasc Interv 2011;4:344–6.

30. Saeed B, Kandzari D, Agostoni P, et al. Use of drug-eluting stents for chronic total occlusions: a systematic review and meta-analysis. Catheter Cardiovasc Interv 2011;77:315–32.

31. Tanaka H, Kadota K, Hosogi S, et al. Mid-term angiographic and clinical outcomes from antegrade versus retrograde recanalization for chronic total occlusions. J Am Coll Cardiol 2011;57: E1628.

32. Brilakis ES, Banerjee S. Advances in the treatment of coronary artery aneurysms. Catheter Cardiovasc Interv 2011;77:1042–4.

Percutaneous Chronic Total Occlusion Revascularization
Program Development, Resource Utilization, and Economic Outcomes

Dimitri Karmpaliotis, MD[a],*, Nicholas J. Lembo, MD[a],
Emmanouil S. Brilakis, MD, PhD[b], David E. Kandzari, MD[a]

KEYWORDS

- Chronic total occlusion • Revascularization • Resource utilization
- Percutaneous coronary intervention

KEY POINTS

- Introduce the concept of the chronic total occlusion (CTO) team rather than focus on individual operator training alone as an essential strategy for successful, safe, and efficient CTO percutaneous coronary intervention (PCI).
- Understand the issues related to resource utilization for CTO PCI and recognize hospital settings in which CTO PCI may economically contribute to positive contribution margins.
- Essential to the initiation of a CTO program is the consensus among cardiologists and hospital administrators regarding the rationale for CTO revascularization.
- Appropriate patient selection and individualized consideration of the risk/benefit is crucial.
- Establishment of a quality assurance program with accountability of technical (including radiation dose) procedural results and acute and long-term clinical outcomes is an opportunity for standardizing protocols and implementing changes.

INTRODUCTION

Despite their prevalence in 20% to 30% of patients with coronary artery disease identified by angiography,[1] chronic total occlusions (CTOs) remain the most common reason for referral to surgical revascularization or relegation to medical therapy.[2] The presence of a CTO has been associated with incomplete revascularization among individuals with multivessel coronary disease, reduced survival, and impaired self-assessed quality of life.[3–5] Denoted as the "last barrier to PCI success," the frequency of attempted percutaneous CTO revascularization, balanced by the perception of a high procedural complication risk and uncertainty of the outcome, remains disappointingly low; despite treatment bias, historical rates of procedural and technical success remain stagnant.[2] There is accumulating evidence that successful percutaneous CTO revascularization, particularly in patients with left ventricular dysfunction, left anterior descending artery as the target vessel, or large ischemic burden, is associated with the resolution of angina symptoms,[6,7] improvement in left ventricular systolic function,[8] or enhanced survival.[9–11]

Despite the clinically meaningful benefit associated with percutaneous CTO revascularization,

[a] Piedmont Heart Institute, 275 Collier Road North West, Suite 300, Atlanta, GA 30309, USA; [b] Division of Cardiology, VA North Texas Health Care System, The University of Texas Southwestern Medical Center at Dallas, 4500 South Lancaster Road, Dallas, TX 75216, USA
* Corresponding author.
E-mail address: dimitri.karmpaliotis@piedmont.org

Intervent Cardiol Clin 1 (2012) 391–395
doi:10.1016/j.iccl.2012.04.004

several misperceptions regarding the clinical indication and benefit persist: a chronically occluded artery is considered clinically benign, collateral channels are sufficient for angina relief, and the area subtended by the CTO is not viable; attempted CTO revascularization is associated with an unacceptably high complication rate; skillsets and technique are foreign to North American interventionalists and may not be transferrable to practices with different standards and risk tolerance; and CTO percutaneous coronary intervention (PCI) is an economic disincentive for hospitals. Despite recent evidence to the contrary for each issue, there remains a need to inform clinicians regarding the indications and appropriateness for CTO PCI.

Against the background of current data supporting indications for CTO revascularization and strategies that promote incrementally higher procedural success rates, this article introduces a multidisciplinary approach to CTO program development, establishes guidelines for performance of safe and efficient CTO PCI and reviews considerations related to resource utilization and economic outcomes with complex percutaneous coronary revascularization.

RATIONALE AND DESIGN OF A CTO PROGRAM

The consensus decision among cardiologists (both noninvasive and interventional) and hospital administrators regarding the clinical rationale for CTO revascularization, appropriate patient identification, and individualized consideration of the risk/benefit is essential to the initiation of a CTO program. Hospital administrators should acknowledge and support the clinical merit (and regional/national recognition) for referral of a patient population often without a therapeutic alternative. Financial administrators should prepare for greater resource utilization and costs but may also forecast similar contribution margins to those on non-CTO cases and overall greater catheterization laboratory volume.

Informing hospital and catheterization laboratory administrators of the CTO initiative's outcomes is also important to ensuring the advancement of the program. As an example, the establishment of a quality assurance program with detailed accountability of technical and procedural results, in-hospital outcomes, and late-term clinical follow-up represents an opportunity for standardizing protocols and systematically implementing changes. The education of catheterization laboratory nurses and technicians, both through didactic and practical training, is also required.

The identification of volunteered operators with the interest and commitment for dedicated and ongoing training in CTO PCI is essential to the CTO team concept. Depending on the interventional volume of the center, having more than one CTO operator involved is likely to expedite the learning curve and also assist in other aspects of program development, such as educating colleagues and referring physicians. Attending regional, national, and international CTO meetings and workshops, as well as participating in Internet-based training activities and events (eg, www.ctofundamentals.org) is strongly encouraged, but there is no substitute for engaging in a proctor/mentor relationship with an expert operator.[12] Educating and engaging catheterization laboratory technicians and nurses is an integral part of the process. In particular, setting expectations for staff is especially relevant. CTO PCI can be time consuming and involves the application of interventional techniques that are counterintuitive compared with non-CTO PCI. Equipment utilization may also be unfamiliar to even experienced interventionalists and staff. Further, unlike the treatment of less complex coronary disease, CTO PCI is associated with a higher incidence of procedural failure and complications that are more unique to CTO PCI. Accordingly, a well-educated and motivated catheterization laboratory team and floor supporting staff is critical for the success of the program.

CTO PROGRAM GUIDELINES

A fundamental aspect of CTO PCI is a patient-focused assessment of procedural appropriateness and risk/benefit assessment. The establishment of routine CTO team meetings to prospectively review indication and procedural strategy informs both the interventional team and the informed consent process. For these reasons, performance of ad hoc CTO PCI is strongly discouraged. The analysis of prior cases also permits peer review and ensures adherence to quality initiatives. The development of a CTO database is also encouraged to permit internal review of the outcomes, identify deviations from program guidelines, and systematically detail the learning curve of CTO PCI success.

A 2-operator-per-case policy (1 primary, 1 assistant) is proposed, which broadens operator exposure and permits collaborative discussion of strategy during the procedure. In addition, a dedicated CTO day should be reserved each week for scheduling CTO cases to give CTO PCI advanced preparation, minimal interruption, and no interference with the remainder of the catheterization laboratory schedule and case flow.

Informed Consent

A review by the CTO interventionalist, with patients and their families, of the procedural risk and benefit, estimate of outcome, and treatment alternatives is mandatory. An explanation of the risk for complications associated with complex coronary revascularization, including contrast nephropathy, radiation dermatitis, and vascular injury (eg, perforation), not only details the risk but also provides patients with an understanding of the procedural complexity. Further, the estimation of the likelihood for procedural success assists in setting expectations in instances of procedural failure. In parallel, an explanation of the methods used to prevent complications (eg, preprocedural hydration, minimizing radiation exposure) offers patient reassurance. In all instances, a general discussion regarding treatment plans and expectations in the event of both a successful (eg, dual antiplatelet therapy adherence) and unsuccessful outcome (eg, planned second attempt, advancement of medical therapy) is suggested before the CTO procedure.

Contrast and Radiation Exposure

Before a CTO program initiation, collaboration between the interventionalists and hospital radiation safety experts is useful to adopt imaging techniques that minimize radiation exposure to patients and laboratory personnel. Guidelines regarding maximum limits of radiation exposure per case and postprocedure follow-up of patients in cases of significant radiation exposure should be established (**Box 1**). Because thresholds for maximum the radiation dose and what criteria constitute a sentinel event vary according to state, each program should establish local standards after a consultation with the hospital radiation safety experts.

Similarly, the adherence to guidelines for the prevention of contrast nephropathy and postprocedural surveillance of patients receiving large contrast volumes is relevant to CTO PCI (see **Box 1**). In selected instances, the risk of contrast-induced kidney injury may exceed the clinical benefit.

Procedural Protocol

CTO PCI cases may be technically challenging and demand an unusually high level of attention and focus from the operator. Although uncommon, operator fatigue should be recognized in instances of prolonged procedures, and termination of the case should be considered.

Unfractionated heparin is the preferred antithrombin therapy given the potential to monitor

---

Box 1
Program guidelines related to radiation exposure, contrast utilization, and antithrombotic monitoring during CTO percutaneous revascularization

Radiation Exposure

Collaborate with institutional radiation safety personnel.

Adopt imaging techniques to minimize radiation dose (*eg*, collimation, field of magnification, alternating view angulation).

Abort procedure if (1) a lesion is not crossed by 8 Gy and (2) the dose reaches 12 Gy at any time.

Provide radiation counseling for every patient receiving greater than or equal to 60 minutes of fluoroscopy time or 6 Gy exposures.

Educate patients at discharge regarding symptoms and signs of radiation injury and instructions to contact the treating physician.

In the absence of a skin injury, delay repeat procedures for at least 60 days unless emergency indication.

In the presence of a prior skin injury, consider any repeat procedures only after a consultation with experts (radiation physicists, dermatologists, plastic surgeons).

Iodinated Contrast Exposure

Adopt techniques to minimize contrast use (dilution of dye, use wires for markers, intravascular ultrasound, and so forth).

Counsel patients who receive more than 5 mL × Kg/creatinine of contrast and obtain chemistry laboratory studies the day following the procedure and 5 days after discharge (results will be communicated [eg, fax to the CTO operator]).

Maintain a higher threshold to perform CTO PCI in patients with compromised renal function.

Adhere to the standard preprocedure and postprocedure renal protective therapies relevant to all complex PCI cases (eg, saline hydration, bicarbonate, discontinuing nephrotoxic medications).

---

the degree of anticoagulation during extended procedures and reverse the anticoagulant effect with protamine in uncommon instances of perforation. The monitoring and documentation of anticoagulation during the procedure is imperative, and the interventional team should be alerted every 30 minutes by a set timer; the activated clotting time (ACT) is maintained between 250 to 300 seconds for antegrade CTO revascularization and approximately 300 to 350 seconds for retrograde procedures.

Simultaneous with the documentation of the ACT, the radiation dose (air kerma) and contrast volume should be verbally reported to the CTO team and recorded. Acknowledgment by the interventionalists is mandatory because it provides a routine standardized update to inform clinical decision making regarding anticoagulant therapy, methods to reduce contrast and radiation exposure, changing procedural strategy, or even terminating the case.

PROCEDURAL, IN-HOSPITAL, AND ECONOMIC OUTCOMES

As an example of implementing a CTO program according to the previously described methods, the authors recently reported a prospective analysis of procedural and early clinical outcomes following attempted CTO revascularization.[13] Among 145 patients, 160 consecutive CTO revascularization procedures were attempted between October 2009 and December 2010. Selected procedural and technical characteristics included bilateral femoral access (90.0%), planned retrograde guidewire placement (37.5%), and reattempted CTO procedure (10.6%). Total procedural fluoroscopic time was (mean ± standard deviation) 67.4 ± 45.5 minutes, and contrast volume was 403 ± 215 mL. The average stent number and the total stent length per CTO vessel were 2.6 ± 1.1 and 64.7 ± 30.7 respectively. The overall CTO success rate was 85.6% (137/160). In-hospital adverse outcomes included death (0.6%), emergency bypass surgery (0.6%), tamponade (0.6%), myocardial infarction (1.9%), and transient nephropathy (1.2%). Altogether, the results suggest that the requirement of educational and performance standards, mentorship from experts, consensus review for appropriateness, and provision of catheterization laboratory policies may represent a model for program development. Moreover, following program-specific quality and performance guidelines, complex CTO revascularization may be safely performed with outcomes comparable to reports from more established centers.[14–18]

CTO REVASCULARIZATION: ECONOMIC DISINCENTIVE OR ATTRACTION?

Because CTO revascularization is often associated with greater equipment utilization and catheterization laboratory time, CTO PCI has been misrepresented as an economic disincentive.[2] Such references are largely without basis given that limited data exist regarding the cost-related metrics and resource utilization associated with these complex and time-consuming procedures;

furthermore, it is unknown in which hospital settings CTO PCI may be economically favorable.

To address these uncertainties, the authors examined resource utilization and hospital contribution margins associated with CTO PCI and non-CTO PCI.[13] Total charges, payments, and direct costs per patient were assessed for 154 CTO procedures and compared with 1847 elective non-CTO PCI cases performed over the same time interval. Among the non-CTO cohort, the average stent utilization was significantly lower (1.4 ± 0.88 non-CTO vs 2.5 ± 1.5 CTO, P<.0001), yet mean hospital stay duration did not significantly differ (2.3 ± 3.2 non-CTO vs 1.9 ± 3.4 CTO, P = .36). Compared with the non-CTO group, CTO PCI was associated with significantly higher charges and reimbursement per patient. Specifically, procedural supply costs were more than twice those related to less complex procedures ($6230 vs $3060, P<.001), driven largely by greater use of balloon angioplasty catheters, guidewires, and coronary stents. Total procedural time (ie, catheterization laboratory utilization time) was additionally 2-fold higher with CTO procedures (2.9 ± 1.3 hours vs 1.3 ± 0.7 hours, P<.0001). djusting for costs related to catheterization laboratory utilization and additional in-hospital non–procedural-related expenses, total direct costs were also higher among CTO procedures ($10,870 vs $7436, P<.001). Despite the higher direct costs, the contribution margin per patient for CTO revascularization remained positive because of the increased total charges and reimbursement and did not statistically vary compared with non-CTO PCI ($5173 vs $5730 P = .58). Accordingly, despite higher resource utilization, CTO revascularization is associated with a positive contribution margin.

SUMMARY

Trainingfor CTO PCI requires considerable commitment from operators and institutional investment in resources, and the need for establishing a model of care delivery and quality assurance at individual centers is fundamental to program success. Through the systematic adoption of complex procedural techniques and adherence to quality oversight, a multiple-operator, high-volume CTO interventional program is achievable with outcomes that exceed historical standards and that are comparable to contemporary reports from international centers with established experience. Specifically, CTO PCI may be performed safely and with high procedural and clinical success through (1) both on- and off-site didactic training and proctoring, (2) adoption of advanced technique and device technology in carefully selected cases, (3) provision of catheterization laboratory policies, and

(4) inclusion of all outcomes as part of a quality and performance initiative. Although once considered a labor- and resource-intensive procedure whose costs exceeded reimbursement, CTO PCI is instead associated with a positive hospital contribution margin similar to less complex PCI. These recent data, therefore, indicate that CTO revascularization should not be considered an economic deterrent, at least in centers with multiple catheterization laboratories that permit dedicated time for such procedures. Altogether, requirement of educational and performance standards, consensus review for appropriateness, attention to cost and resource utilization, and provision of catheterization laboratory guidelines represents a model for CTO program development that may be extended to other complex percutaneous revascularization indications.

REFERENCES

1. Stone GW, Kandzari DE, Mehran R, et al. Percutaneous recanalization of chronically occluded coronary arteries: a consensus document: part I. Circulation 2005;112: 2364–72.
2. Grantham JA, Marso SP, Spertus J, et al. Chronic total occlusion angioplasty in the United States. JACC Cardiovasc Interv 2009;2:479–86.
3. Valenti R, Migliorini A, Signorini U, et al. Impact of complete revascularization with percutaneous coronary intervention on survival in patients with at least one chronic total occlusion. Eur Heart J 2008;29:2336–42.
4. Hanna EL, Racz M, Holmes DR, et al. Impact of completeness of percutaneous coronary intervention revascularization on long-term outcomes in the stent era. Circulation 2006;113:2406–12.
5. Grantham JA, Jone PG, Cannon L, et al. Quantifying the early health status benefits of successful chronic total occlusion recanalization: results from the FlowCardia's Approach to Chronic Total Occlusion recanalization (FACTOR) trial. Circ Cardiovasc Qual Outcomes 2010;3(3):284–90.
6. Ivanohe RJ, Weintraub WS, Douglas JS Jr, et al. Percutaneous transluminal coronary angioplasty of chronic total occlusions. Primary success, restenosis, and long-term clinical follow-up. Circulation 1992;85:106–15.
7. Olivari Z, Rubartelli P, Piscione F, et al. Immediate results and one-year clinical outcome after percutaneous coronary interventions in chronic total occlusions: data from a multi-center, prospective, observational study (TOAST-GISE). J Am Coll Cardiol 2003;41:1672–8.
8. Kirschbaum SW, Baks T, van den Ent M, et al. Evaluation of left ventricular function three years after percutaneous recanalization of chronic total occlusions. Am J Cardiol 2008;101:179–85.
9. Joyal D, Afilalo J, Rinfret S. Effectiveness of recanalization of chronic total occlusions: a systematic review and meta-analysis. Am Heart J 2010;160: 179–87.
10. Mehran R, Claessen BE, Godino C, et al. Long-term outcome of percutaneous coronary intervention for chronic total occlusions. JACC Cardiovasc Interv 2011;4:952–61.
11. Safley DM, House JA, Marso SP, et al. Improvement in survival following successful percutaneous coronary intervention of coronary chronic total occlusions: variability by target vessel. JACC Cardiovasc Interv 2008; 1:295–302.
12. Di Mario C, Werner GS, Sianos G, et al. European perspective in the recanalisation of chronic total occlusions (CTO): consensus document from the EuroCTO club. EuroIntervention 2007;3:30–43.
13. Karmpaliotis D, Lembo N, Kalynych A, et al. Development of a high-volume, multiple-operator program for percutaneous chronic total coronary occlusion revascularization: procedural, clinical and cost-utilization outcomes. Cathet Cardiovasc Interv, in press.
14. Rathore S, Matsuo H, Terashima M, et al. Procedural and in-hospital outcomes after percutaneous coronary intervention for chronic total occlusions of coronary arteries 2002 to 2008. Impact of novel guidewire techniques. JACC Cardiovasc Interv 2009;2:489–97.
15. Morino Y, Kimura T, Hayashi Y, et al. In-hospital outcomes of contemporary percutaneous coronary intervention in patients with chronic total occlusion. Insights from the J-CTO Registry (Multicenter CTO Registry of Japan). JACC Cardiovasc Interv 2010; 3:143–51.
16. Galassi AR, Tomasello SD, Reifart N, et al. In-hospital outcomes of percutaneous coronary intervention in patients with chronic total occlusion: insights from the ERCTO (European Registry of Chronic Total Occlusion) registry. EuroIntervention 2011;7:472–9.
17. Thompson CA, Jayne JE, Robb JF, et al. Retrograde techniques and the impact of operator volume on percutaneous intervention for coronary chronic total occlusions: an early United States experience. JACC Cardiovasc Interv 2009;2:834–42.
18. Kandzari DE. Import and export of interventional technique: something to declare at the border. JACC Cardiovasc Interv 2009;2:843–5.

Index

Note: Page numbers of article titles are in **boldface** type.

Intervent Cardiol Clin 1 (2012) 397–400
http://dx.doi.org/10.1016/S2211-7458(12)00085-5
2211-7458/12/$ – see front matter © 2012 Elsevier Inc. All rights reserved.

interventional.theclinics.com

Printed and bound by CPI Group (UK) Ltd, Croydon, CR0 4YY

03/10/2024

01040361-0020

Moving?

Make sure your subscription moves with you!

To notify us of your new address, find your **Clinics Account Number** (located on your mailing label above your name), and contact customer service at:

Email: journalscustomerservice-usa@elsevier.com

800-654-2452 (subscribers in the U.S. & Canada)
314-447-8871 (subscribers outside of the U.S. & Canada)

Fax number: 314-447-8029

Elsevier Health Sciences Division
Subscription Customer Service
3251 Riverport Lane
Maryland Heights, MO 63043

*To ensure uninterrupted delivery of your subscription, please notify us at least 4 weeks in advance of move.

ELSEVIER